COMBATTING NEGATIVE MINDSET

Manual for Success

COMBATTING NEGATIVE MINDSET

Manual for Success

Jongikhaya Siwali

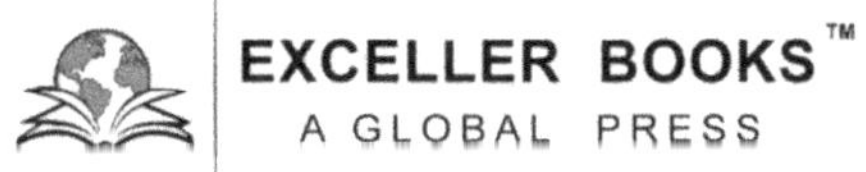

Combatting Negative Mindset
Manual for Success

ISBN: 978-81-19524-70-9

First published in India in 2024 by Exceller Books,
An Imprint of GE Group

Address: G1, Dream Apartment, Degree College Road, Belgharia, Kolkata, 700056, India

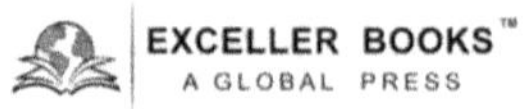

EXCELLER BOOKS™
A GLOBAL PRESS

https://excellerbooks.com/

Dedication

To the people who have influenced my life:

My late Pastor S. Dayi, who pastored me; Rev. P. Mabhena, my probation mentor; the late Rev. Nkuhlu, for the brief moments we shared; and many others who touched my broken life and family. Lastly, to my immediate family, who brought a new dawn into my life.

This message is for all who shaped me, through both good and bad experiences. I thank the Lord for you all.

Thank you.

Acknowledgements

Sponsors and donors who believed in the process of change, and schools that wanted to adopt and try this program, have all played a crucial role. Influencers in my work as a Youth Worker, Church Pastor, Teacher, and Chaplain have also contributed significantly. These influences helped me believe there is a way to reach children who are indifferent to their development and do not appreciate teachers and parents who want the best for them.

The students from Khulani Commercial High School expressed their appreciation to me on the street, thanking me for including this program in their lives and acknowledging the difference it made.

My wife Pumeza, and my children Kamva and Sine, gave meaning to my contributions to the lives of others. Their love and appreciation inspired me to want the same for others. Our NPO was named after them and reflects God's will for us as Jongikhaya Siwalis.

I bless and thank everyone who contributed to the possibility of this program and the writing of this manual, whether knowingly or unknowingly.

Table of Contents

Module I:
Introduction

Session 1: Setting the Scene

AIM, OBJECTIVES, AND OUTLINE

Note to Facilitator. The program starts with this session, which sets the scene. In this session, the participant learns what to expect from the program.

Session Aim. By the end of this session, participants will start to know each other, begin group formation, and understand what the course wants to address.

Session Objectives. By the end of this session, participants will be able to:
   a) Describe the aim and objectives of the program.
   b) Describe the method that will be followed.
   c) Identify the ground rules that the group has set for the course.

Session Outline
   a) Starting the session
   b) Introducing all participants
   c) Establishing ground rules
   d) Importance the course
   e) Course Overview
   f) Hod
   g) Personal Action Plan

PREPARATION

Preparation by Facilitator

<u>Prepare the Training Venue</u>
a) Facilitators should meet at least one hour before the time to finalize all
b) Last-minute arrangements and address organizational issues.
c) Prepare nametags for all participants.
d) Prepare an Attendance List.
e) Prepare copies of the programme for all members.

Preparation by Participants
None

MATERIALS AND EQUIPMENT
a) Slideshow: Slide on:
b) Aim
c) Name Tags
d) Scope Method
e) Outcomes of Programme
f) Table of Contents
    i. Write the Table of Contents neatly on a Flip Chart and paste it on the wall.
    ii. Make Copies of the Personal Data Sheet (Appendix C) for each participant to fill in.
    iii. Compile an attendance list with your name, surname, and contact number.
    iv. Do an ice-breaker and ask where they grew up and share something that nobody else in the room. Already knows about them.

ITEM 1.2: ESTABLISHING GROUND RULES

(10 Minutes)

Facilitate the ground rules for the week. Write agreed-upon ground rules on a flip chart. If it does not come from the group, add the following:
   a) Cell phones off.
   b) Punctuality.
   c) Viewpoints respected.

Appoint a timekeeper and a person to handle the evaluation forms after each session.

ITEM 1.3: IMPORTANCE OF THE COURSE

(5 Minutes)

Emphasize the importance of the course by sharing some of the following with the group:

This course will be one of the most important courses you will ever take. What you learn in this course may literally save your life. In these sessions, we are not going to study an academic subject. Instead, our subject in this class is going to be you and your life. We will talk about the things that are most important to you (your life and the way you live it).

We are going to learn about your hopes and dreams and about some of the decisions you are facing. We are going to talk about how you came to those decisions and whether you have the skills to stick to your decisions. This course will help you make important decisions with consequences for life and death.

We are going to talk about friends, family, relationships, and marriage. You are going to learn many things that will help you to have a happy, exciting, and fulfilling life. We are going to see how you can avoid some of the dangers that might hurt or even destroy your life. This includes the danger of becoming infected by NEGATIVE MINDSET.

You will be examining your own values and will be taught skills that will not only help you to face the threat of a NEGATIVE MINDSET but will also empower you in all walks of life.

ITEM 1.4: COURSE OVERVIEW

(10 Minutes)

Go through the table of content that was beforehand written on a flip chart and pasted on one of the walls and briefly introduce the participants to the main topics that will be covered. A transparency of the table of content can also be used.

ITEM 1.5: METHOD

Tell the following to the group:
This course will make use of a participatory learning approach. Participants will all contribute and learn from each other. We, the course leaders, will be facilitators, helping you to discover what you want to know. Your views will be incorporated into the learning process. At all times, your beliefs will be respected. No decision or choices will be forced on you. This, however, does not mean that your views will not be challenged.

ITEM 1.6: PERSONAL ACTION PLAN

(3 Minutes)

In Appendix A of the course material, there is a personal commitment sheet. During the course, you will regularly be given the opportunity to write about things that you would like to change in your lifestyle. At the end of the course, you will be afforded the opportunity to make a pledge, committing yourself to an improved value-based lifestyle.

Session 2: Severity of Negative Mindset

AIM, OBJECTIVES, AND OUTLINE

Note to Facilitator. Although all people function from a specific value Mindset, most people are unaware of the influence that mindset has on their actions. This session aims to introduce the participants to their own mindset and belief system. An introduction is given to what is understood under the term "mindset". The participant is then also introduced to mindset-frameworks and the discovering of his/her own mindset.

Session Aim. By the end of this session, participants will understand the importance of addressing a NEGATIVE MINDSET prevention program.

Session Objectives. By the end of this session, participants will be able to:
   a) Describe the meaning and importance of mindset and mindset frame frameworks.
   b) Describe the mindset framework of this course.
   c) Describe what their own mindset framework is.
   d) Describe the implications of mindset for living.
   e) Describe the link between mindset and religion.
   f) Describe the link between mindset, values and culture.
   g) Explore some of the group's norms and customs that have an influence on NEGATIVE MINDSET prevention.

Session Outline

Discuss

Mindset and how they influence our lives	35 minutes
The Mindset framework of this course	18 minutes
Personal Action Plan	3 minutes
Important or not important customs?	40 minutes
Religion and Values.	20 minutes
Cultural values and NEGATIVE MINDSET	25 minutes
Conclusion	10 minutes
Intro next session	3 minutes
Total Time	144 minutes

PREPARATION

Preparation by Facilitator
Prepare slide show.

Preparation by Participants
None

MATERIALS AND EQUIPMENT

Slideshow: dumping, slums, filthiness, drugs, teen problems, etc.
Definition of Ubuntu.

Session 3: Introducing Values

AIM, OBJECTIVES, AND OUTLINE

Note to Facilitator. Although all people function from a specific value system, most people are unaware of the influence that values have on their actions. This session wants to introduce the participants to their own values and belief systems. An introduction is given to what is understood under the term "values". The participant is then also introduced to value-frameworks and the discovering of his/her own values.

Session Aim. By the end of this session, participants will understand the importance of addressing values in a NEGATIVE MINDSET prevention program.

Session Objectives. By the end of this session, participants will be able to:

a) Describe the meaning and importance of values and value frameworks.
b) Describe the value framework of this course.
c) Describe what their own value framework is.
d) Describe the implications of values for living.
e) Describe the link between values and religion.
f) Describe the link between values and culture.
g) Explore some of the group's norms and customs that have an influence on NEGATIVE MINDSET prevention.

Session 4: Self-Identity

Objectives

To communicate that man works well in synergy, unity of spirit, mind and body. What man does not have in spirit and mind cannot manifest in the physic. Success depends on a healthy spirit and brain.

Aim

To help students to learn that spirituality and ethics go with success. Life with discipline is easy form to achieve desired lifestyle.

Appendix B: Questionnaire: Discovering Your Identity

AIM, OBJECTIVES, AND OUTLINE

Note to Facilitator. In order to combat NEGATIVE MINDSET, it is necessary to know who you are and what your dreams and viewpoints are. Therefore, this session is designed for the Participants to discover their own identity. In this session, the participants must continue to discover their values. They cannot protect their values with assertiveness if they do not know their values. They must also be made aware of their dreams that form part of their self-identity. These dreams are threatened if they are not able to protect them with value based decisions and assertiveness.

Session Aim. By the end of this session, participants will be able to identify who they are and the implications of NEGATIVE

MINDSET on their dreams for the future.

Session Objectives. By the end of this session, participants will be able to:

a)   List the things that they think make them unique.

b)   List their dreams for the future.

c)   Determine the influence of NEGATIVE MINDSET infection on those dreams.

Session Outline

Ice Breaker: From Animal World	10 minutes
Questionnaire: Discover your identity	20 minutes
Where do I want to be in 20 years?	10 minutes
How can a NEGATIVE MINDSET influence my dreams?	15 minutes
Personal Action Plan	3 minutes
Conclusion	3 minutes
Total Time	61 minutes

PREPARATION

Preparation by Facilitator
None

Preparation by Participants
None

MATERIALS AND EQUIPMENT
Copies of the questionnaire (Appendix B)

ITEM 4.1: ICE-BREAKER: ANIMAL WORLD

(10 Minutes)

Request all the participants to close their eyes. Ask them the following:

Imagine yourself in an animal world. See all the animals. Pick one that you can imagine you are, and that depicts your characteristics.

Let each participant pair off with another person and explain to that person why they have chosen that particular animal. Thereafter, the participants were asked to share their choices with the larger group.

Tell the group that this exercise demonstrates differences in identity. We are all unique people.

ITEM 4-2: QUESTIONNAIRE: DISCOVER YOUR INDIVIDUAL IDENTITY (Exercise 7)

(20 Minutes)

Give every participant an individual questionnaire. This will help them discover their own identity. This questionnaire deals with:

a) What are the *setbacks* that I had in life?

b) What were the things that helped me to *cope* with my setbacks?

c) What are the *strengths* of my personality?

d) What are the *weaknesses* in my personality?

c) How do other people perceive me?

f) How do I want to be? I dream of...

g) How does God perceive me?

h) What are my personal *values?* (The way you really spend your time and resources is a very good indicator of what you truly value.)

i)   What do I stand for, and what do I believe in?

After they have filled in the questionnaire, have them draw a rough sketch of a tree that represents their life. Let the roots represent the things/persons from which they draw their strength, the trunk be the things that enable them to cope, the branches their unique quality (strengths and weaknesses), and the leaves and fruit be things which they have achieved and what they are busy achieving. Draw a few branches that broke off. This represents setbacks. Make them aware that, despite the setbacks, the tree is living and growing, and they hope to be still vibrant, a place to come.

Divide the participants in a group of two and let them share with the other person what they discovered about themselves and their Identity. Tell the group about the things they have written down and the pictures they have drawn. They are proof of their identity, who they are, where they come from, and whether it is what they dream of. Then, ask them to think of moments with the following question:

EXERCISE: 8

(10 Minutes)

On a piece of paper, draw five columns. Write down one thing in each column that you would like to accomplish in the next twenty years.

In 3 years	In 5 years	In 8 years	In 20 years

End off by Saying:

The wonderful thing about life is that we have choices and also the choice of who we want to be. What you put into life is what you will get out of life. Let us inspire ourselves with the slogan: "If you can dream it, you can achieve it if you aim for these goals – put blinkers on and go for it! Believe in yourself – your talents, skills and abilities.

ITEM 4-4: HOW CAN NEGATIVE MINDSET-INFECTION INFLUENCE MY DREAMS? (Exercise 9)

(15 Minutes)

Let all participants answer the following questions on a piece of paper for themselves:

a) What implications will it have for me as a person if I go for a NEGATIVE MINDSET
b) How can a NEGATIVE MINDSET infection influence my dreams for the future?
c) What can I do to protect myself and my dreams?

ITEM 4-5: PERSONAL ACTION PLAN

(3 Minutes)

Write down in the space next to question 3 on your personal commitment sheet what you intend to do in future to increase your level of being true to yourself, who you are and where you want to go with your life.

ITEM 4-6: CONCLUSION

Conclude by saying:

We are all unique human beings. My identity is who I was, who I um, und who I wlll be. NEGATIVE MINDSET is a threat to our existence and our dreams. If a sound value system is part of our identity, the risk of getting infected is much smaller. Therefore, make sure you know which values and convictions are part of your identity, and then say to yourself: Because I know who I am and what I believe, I want to follow the values that I believe.

In the following sessions, we are going to address the specific values that we think are important to combating the threat of NEGATIVE MINDSET. The values are:

a) Love.
b) Responsibility
c) Fairness.
d) Integrity (including trust and loyalty).
e) Respect.
f) Professionalism

Identity Explained

The identity of a person is seen in many things: *who* he is, *what* he is, and *why* she is. Talking about what mankind is the description, he gets on how he existed and the purpose thereof. Religion as a Spirit will play a big role in this and, therefore, also set up some standards of who mankind should be. Again, as a Soul, the capabilities he possesses intellectually and in interaction with the universe are the creativity of the entire universal mind and his individual mental capability to achieve amongst the others and as part of his community/ society. Then there is a bio, the physical man in the physical world.

Discuss

Mankind is the spiritual entity; what is the Identity?
Mankind as the Psyche, Psychological entity; what is the Identity?
Mankind as the Bios, Physical entity; what is the Identity?

Discuss

How everyone would love to be known and if they would like to be remembered and how; when old and they died: how would you like your children to write on your tombstone?

Module: II
Foundation of Success Mindset

Session 5: Foundation

Foundation Explained

This is a term also used in or when doing construction work. This means a structure needs to stand on underbuilt platform structure. The structure of the unseen that will affect strength on what is seen. Usually, the foundation is built but it is not seen. The seen part is based on that which is not seen.

How big and strong the seen structure should be is always based on how big and strong that which is unseen structure is underneath.

The foundation is designed by engineers: the drawing by architect, work by qualified artisans. Three spheres of that cannot be interchanged to do each other's job.

In the same manner, the life of an individual or community is built upon this principle. Let me tell you that each and every one of us has a lot of work to do if we are going to be building our lives. Lots of unseen work, a lot of planning work and a lot of Implementation work.

They need to first build from the unseen (unconscious) to the subconscious to the conscious. Spirit, Soul (mind), and Physical.

Unconscious Mind

Out there is the Unseen World of every possibility and promise of life, good and evil, that we discover every day. Just the other, they discovered that there are more planets than we had known. They discovered that there are laws that govern nature and the supernatural. They discovered that we can make electricity, discovered waves for communication, and discovered that a big object can fly in the sky and many more. That removes a canopy of sceptics, doubt, fear, unbelief and disbelief. There is now no limitation to what is possible in life, and it cannot be limited by the skies anymore, not even the universe; there is a possibility of what is higher than the Sky and universe; there is a possibility of a God and higher systems out there. This means that a vast amount of what is not known yet is waiting to be discovered. It places humans to become great scientists, the type we have not seen yet, great Spiritism that has not been seen yet and great biologists that have not been seen yet. What is exciting is that you are part of that; it's just that you do not know.

Subconscious Mind

The knowledge that has been discovered and is operational lies in books, people's minds and computers, knowledge from the senses and discoveries that can be awakened and that which makes who we are today. Do you know that only humans are entrusted with such information? Data that sometimes works automatically in our systems and the ecosystem that we interact with. It affects people individually, including families, communities, and societies. This, at times, happens whether we believe it or not, know it or not, feel it or not, etc.

Conscious Mind

This is what is available to you clear and not so clear, creating the reality of the existence of things. To qualify the brain. The brain is the whole body and senses. The mind coexists with the brain, feeding it with outer spheres of life. The existing, the under buried, and the unknown are yet to be known. Consciousness is what is already revealed and known to you.

The fact is it is impossible for anyone not to believe that there is vast of the unknown out there. It is a fact people that have been successful they have stepped into that sphere. So when you are asked about the existence of God, it is a question that deeply asks you about the deep understanding of the unconscious mind. How connected are you with the world of the unseen.

Discussion

What does that mean for you?
How do you build yourself to build mental capacity?
How would you arrive at the reality of your mental dream?

Rubber Hit the Road

Do you have dreams: do you believe in dreams?

Balancing Your Life

Spiritual (Zoe), Mental (Psyche) and matter (Bios)
We fix that which is broken spiritually or create a spirituality that will enable you to grow mentally and then be on construction till you become.

Session 6: Maslow's Pyramid of Needs

Kunjani Mnganam?

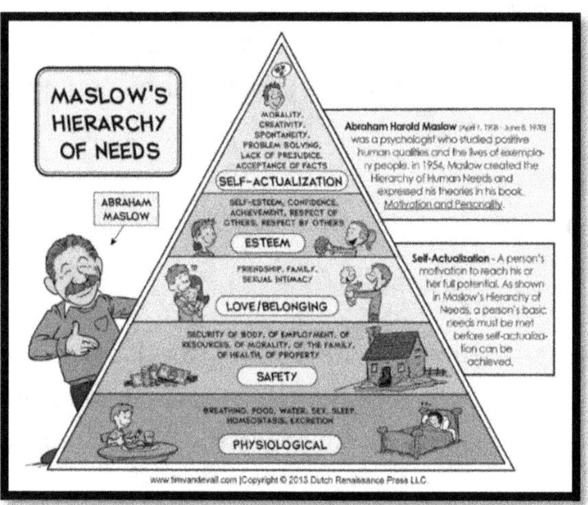

The hierarchy needs to be seen with the eyes of grading and ratings. Competition of life, not a ladder

  i.   The question is where am I in the race life?
    a)   Physiological
    b)   Safety-wise:
    c)   Love and belonging:
    d)   Esteem:
    e)   Self-actualization:
  ii.   Compare to the best nations in the world: where are we in the race
    a)   1st world countries
    b)   2nd world, countries

    c)   3rd world countries

iii.   Discussion: Bantu people will ask you this question: Kunjani?

Kunjani is a simple question, but it seeks to find out how one is coping with the process of life or the competition of life. The question is about actualizing; where are you about actualizing a better person you could be?

Session 7: Teen Road: Balanced Growth

This topic sounds like a tin road: What if the road was made of Tin?

What would it be like? First it would be brilliant and shiny but later turn to rusted and ugly.

Teenage years are very good days for a human being, these are the years of growth where we see ourselves developing to height, beauty, body, knowledge, and spirituality.

Body Development

Puberty growth

Meaning: Sexual decision to make

Psychological Development

Mental growth

Meaning: Career decisions and morality

Spirit Development

Spiritual development

Meaning: God-related decisions

Discussion

Immaturity Signs

Teen pregnancy, drug and substance problems, dropping out, disruptions of school learning, and not being helpful at home. Etc.

What could be the solution?

It is predictable because we have examples right in front of us:

our older brothers and sisters, our parents.

Advice: Spiritual development, Psychological (mindset), and Physical health.

Find yourself a spiritual home:

Find yourself a healthy mindset: abstain from sexual activities; it's not for kings!

Physical health: Avoid teen pregnancy, STD, abortion, drugs, and alcohol. Etc.

Session 8: Mindset

Definition

Mindset is a habitual or a characteristic mental attitude that determines how you are to respond or interpret a situation. This is a very crucial process of thinking and it needs to be developed to give you quality of life and enhance the development of your environment. Mindset if not in good standing can assist all negatives of your life and assist every bewitchment by the negative life.

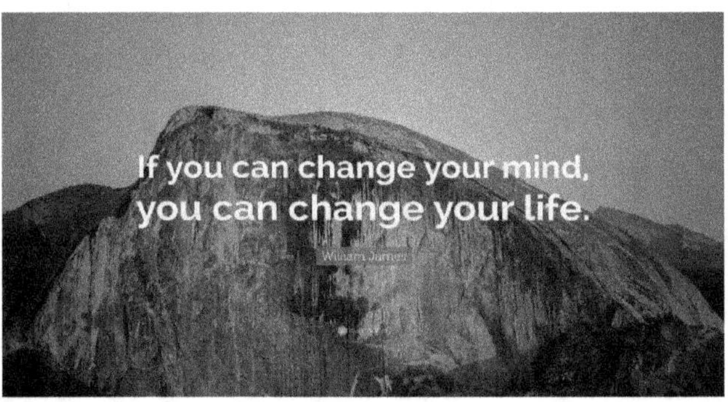

Transformation Is Based on Mindset

Mindset is about setting the mind; the mind comes in sets, and every set will bring you to a sphere or field of thinking. The mindset is the reality of the brain's capacity and fields. This is then projected in life scenarios, which then depicts goodness and evil that you are to interact with in life. The mindset can be projected on what people do.

Music, Image, environment, self, cleanliness, drawings, food, drinks, drugs, etc.

e.g.

A poverty mindset is a way of **thinking** that makes you **believe** that you are poor and will never have enough of anything, especially money. It can be caused by your **thoughts or feelings** about your situation, and it can prevent you from **achieving your goals or building wealth**. A poverty mindset can also be influenced by your **social context or your negative attitude** towards abundance. It can limit your **growth and potential** and make it hard for you **to attract** what you want.

What you are is because of mindset; what your Environment is BECAUSE OF a mindset.

The biblical word *repent* means *changing one's mindset* to a new one.

You can tell of areas that are sociologically ill by dumping, drains, blockages, rates, dirtiness, etc.

Session 9: Divide and Rule VS Synergy

One of Jeshua Mashiach's famous quotes is, "A kingdom divided on itself shall not stand."

Divide and Rule Game: Formula

Discuss the multiparty state weaknesses if they are divided.

Discuss the community's success if they are divided.

Talk about family divisions and the possibilities of being a successful family.

Talk about the human possibility of living a divided life and wanting to succeed and actualize.

Synergy

SYN-ENERGY: TOGETHER ENERGY: PULLING TOGETHER TO ONE DIRECTION; IF THEY CAN NOT UNDERSTAND ILLUSTRATE: take two students to pull each other using a rope: tell them that is divide and rule. Then, tell them to pull one other student, and the second time, the third student is not to resist walking and working with them. Explain that it is synergy.

Discuss Application

Individual unison (body, mind and spirit)

Discuss the problems of the community: Amapara Robbery.

Discuss the beloved country South Africa's multipartyism.

Module 3
Ethical Values Enhancing a Positive Lifestyle

Session 10: Love

AIM, OBJECTIVES, AND OUTLINE

Note to Facilitator. In the previous session participants have seen how vulnerable they are to HIV-Infection. From this session onwards, the participants are introduced to different values that are important to combating the spread of HIV/AIDS. This session addresses the value of love. In this session, the aim is to make participants aware that there are different perceptions of what love really is. Real love is something different from "Hollywood style of love", as well as "Making love". Real Love includes caring love, where selfishness does not have any place. This caring love is in line with the Golden Rule of "Do unto others as you want to be done unto." If we want to combat the HIV pandemic effectively, we will have to embrace real love in our relationships.

Session Aim. By the end of this session, participants will be able to understand the value of applying love that cares to all relationships.

Session Objectives. By the end of this session participants will be able to:
   a) Describe what unselfishness and caring love are.
   b) Describe the relationship between Ubuntu and selfishness and caring love.
   c) Distinguish love from lust.
   d) Express how adopting the value of caring love can contribute to the preventions of HIV/AIDS.

Session Outline

The Nature of True Love	30 Minutes
Ethical Frameworks and Love	20 Minutes
Love and the prevention of NEGATIVE MINDSET	15 Minutes
Personal Action Plan	3 Minutes
Conclusion	3 Minutes
Total Time	71 Minutes

PREPARATION

Preparation by Facilitator
None

Preparation by Participants
None

MATERIALS AND EQUIPMENT
Flipchart and Kokies

ITEM 5-1: THE NATURE OF TRUE LOVE (Exercise 10)

(30 Minutes)

Say to the group:
Imagine that a friend of yours writes to you for advice.

> *Dear,*
> *Last week I met a man who is very good-looking. He thinks I'm really smart too. We went for a walk together, and after the walk, he kissed me. He's a*

really good kisser, and we kissed for a while. I'm not sure I should have kissed him so soon – I mean, maybe he kisses a lot of ladies, but still, I can't wait to see him again. Do you think I'm in love?

– Laura

Ask the group:
    a)   Do you think this is true love? Support your answer. What do you understand under the term "Love"?
    b)   What would you say is the difference between true love, the "Hollywood example of love" and "making love"?
    c)   How can we distinguish when it is true love and when it is still just fulfilling the sexual wants of a person, even if there is no sexual intercourse?

Use the following ideas to help guide the feedback from the group:
    a)   The "love" in the letter is not much more than just some erotic feelings.
    b)   The old Greeks distinguished between different categories of love:
        i.   Erotic Love (Eros)
        ii.   Platonic Love (Fileo)
        iii.   Unselfish, self-sacrificing, caring love (Agape)
    c)   We cannot always have erotic and platonic love feelings towards everybody, but we can always act with an unselfish, caring attitude towards all people. The Hollywood example of love is often merely lust. "Making love" is in itself a contradiction in terms. Love cannot be made. Love is an attitude and an inner commitment towards other people.
    d)   Real love stays committed to the Golden Rule: "Do unto others as you want to be done unto."

e) The following are important aspects of unselfish, caring love in a relationship:

1. Respect for the other person and for oneself.
2. Enjoyment of the relationship.
3. Fun and a sense of humour about life.
4. Affection demonstrated.
5. Comfortable with a partner having other friends and interests.
6. Patience in allowing the relationship to develop over time.
7. Respect for the partner's Ideas, values, and beliefs.
8. Responsible enough to control my own physical desires.
9. Secure in your partner's love.
10. Foundation of friendship.
11. Honest and open communication.
12. Sensitive to Partner's needs.
13. Never put the other person at risk.

f) The following are important indications of dysfunctional or abusive relationships, which are built not on unselfish love but on "something else "?

1. Not valuing partner's ideas, values, beliefs, and emotions.
2. Relationships become burdensome.
3. Fun and a sense of humour become harder to maintain.
4. Take rather than gives.
5. Prominent jealousy.
6. The pressure is put on a partner to yield to physical desires.
7. Neglect of everyone and everything but partner.
8. Growing neglect of partner.

9. Insensitivity to partner's needs.
10. Domination of one partner by the other (possible violence).
11. Broken promises and lack of trust.
12. Guarded communication.
13. Nagging doubts about the relationship.

In a relationship, which is only built on lust, and not on unselfish love, the emphasis in the relationship may be on courting, cuddling, petting, and not on being a friend for the other, serving the other and needs.

ITEM 5-2: ETHICAL FRAMEWORKS AND LOVE (Exercise 11)
(20 Minutes)

Divide in three groups. Let each group discuss one of the following questions for five minutes and give feedback for five minutes.

a) For what reason would religion put such a high value on love?

b) Is there any relationship between Ubuntu and caring love?

c) How can you apply the value of caring love in your everyday life?

Use the following ideas to help guide the feedback from the group:

a) Religion mostly has to do with a worldview that gives a recipe for the peaceful co-existence of people. Unselfish love promotes just that.

b) There is a close relationship between Ubuntu and caring love. The following are common to both:

  i. That you value the good of the community above self-interest.

  ii. That you strive to help others in the spirit of service.

ITEM 5-3: LOVE AND THE PREVENTION OF NEGATIVE MINDSET
(15 Minutes)

Request the group to divide into pairs and answer the question that follows:

In which way can adopting the value of always acting in caring love towards other people help in combating the spread of a NEGATIVE MINDSET

ITEM 5-4: PERSONAL ACTION PLAN

(3 Minutes)

Write down a personal commitment on a sheet of what you intend to do to increase the level of caring love in your behaviour towards other people.

Will you walk the talk?

ITEM 5-5: CONCLUSION

Conclude by making the following statements:

All people are born into relationships. From your birth you have been in relationship with other people. In African culture the Ubuntu concept says: "We are what we are through other people."

  Love is the foundation for any strong and lasting relationship. Sometimes, we have trouble recognizing love when we see it because of the number of counterfeit loves that the world has to offer.

  A person's want of sex can be mistaken for true love. We have to distinguish between love and a person's want for sex. Love is something more.

  We have discovered today that true love is unselfish, caring love, asking what I can give, and not what I can receive from any relationship. This is the essence of the Golden Rule of "Do unto others as you want them to do unto you ".

To fight NEGATIVE MINDSET/AIDS it is necessary that you adopt this value as a non-negotiable in all your relationships.

In our next Session we are going to address the value of taking responsibility for your actions.

Session 11: Responsibility

AIM, OBJECTIVES, AND OUTLINE

Note to Facilitator. In the previous session we addressed the importance of the value of caring love in the fight against NEGATIVE MINDSET. This session addresses the value of taking responsibility for your deeds. It tries to make participants aware that they must take responsibility for whether they are going to become NEGATIVE MINDSET-infected and are going to contribute to the spread of NEGATIVE MINDSET or being part of those combating NEGATIVE MINDSET.

A responsible person is somebody who takes his and his fellow man's interests seriously. He lives according to the Golden Rule of "Do unto others as you want them to do unto you." Great emphasis must be placed on the fact that a responsible person is a person that takes ownership of his/her behavior and the consequences of that behavior.

Session Aim. By the end of this session, participants will appreciate the importance of taking responsibility.

Session Objectives. By the end of this session, participants will be able to:
   a) Describe what they understand under the term "responsibility".
   b) Give examples of being responsible and irresponsible in their behaviour.
   c) Apply their knowledge of responsible behaviour to prevent a NEGATIVE MINDSET.

Session Outline

The Dice	40 minutes
Brainstorm (Define Responsibility)	30 minutes
The fish and the log	5 minutes
Break	5 minutes.
NEGATIVE MINDSET and responsible behaviour	30 minutes
Personal Action Plan	
Conclusion	

PREPARATION

Preparation by Facilitator

Request two participants beforehand to role-play the scenario given in the case study.

Preparation by Participants

None

MATERIALS AND EQUIPMENT

None

ITEM 11-1: INTRODUCTION

Welcome the participants.

Announce the theme:

In this session we are going to discuss the value of taking responsibility.

ITEM 6-2: THE DICE

Write the numbers one to seven each on a separate piece of paper. Paste the numbers with Prestick in different places in the classroom. Tell the group to divide into seven groups and go and stand at each number. Tell them that you are going to throw a dice. Every time it falls on a number, that group becomes s i c k and must sit out. After the first throw, tell them that they can change numbers if they want. You can even encourage them to go and stand on the number that the dice fell on because it is unlikely that the dice will fall twice on the same number. It is like soldiers believing that a bomb never falls in the same place twice. Throw the dice a few times, every time giving the opportunity to change places. The group will slowly start to realize that the only place to be safe, is no.7 because a dice only has six sides.

Let the group afterwards discuss:
a) What did you experience through this exercise?
b) What lesson can be learnt from this exercise for combating a NEGATIVE MINDSET?
c) What do you think will be the most difficult when you apply the lesson that you have learned from this exercise?

Use the following ideas to help guide the feedback from the groups:
The safest way not to get a NEGATIVE MINDSET is not to participate in high-risk behaviour. Taking chances with a NEGATIVE MINDSET is irresponsible behaviour.

We make our own decisions. We can choose to take responsibility for where we are in terms of vulnerability for NEGATIVE MINDSET infection, or we can be irresponsible and stand a chance to get infected.

During the rest of the course repeat the slogan: *"Stay on No 7"*.

ITEM 11-3: BRAINSTORM THE MEANING OF THE TERM RESPONSIBILITY (Exercise 12)

Divide in two groups: Discuss the following questions for 15 minutes and give feedback for 15 minutes. Ask every participant to think of an object that reminds him/her of the following:

a) Responsible behaviour (e.g., a Bible, key, a blank cheque, a photo of parents, etc.) Let them share it with the rest of the group and say why this specific object reminds them of responsible behaviour.

b) What do you understand under the term "responsibility"?

c) What type of behaviour will reveal that you have/do not have "being responsible" as a personal value? How do you apply to be responsible to everyday life?

d) What relationship do you see between Ubuntu and being responsible? What does Ubuntu's philosophy say about being responsible?

Write the student's feedback on what they understand under the term "responsibility" on a flip chart. Underline important words that were mentioned. Use the following ideas to help guide the feedback from the groups.

a) The word responsibility breaks down into "response" and "ability", which is the ability to choose your response. Responsible people do not blame circumstances, conditions, or conditioning for their behaviour. Their behaviour is a product of their own conscious choice. The freedom to choose brings upon us self-awareness, imagination, conscience, and an independent will, which we can institute to become proactive. It means that as human beings, we are responsible for our own lives.

b) People not taking responsibility are driven by feelings, by circumstances, by conditions, or by their environment. In contrast to these people, we find those who could subordinate such an impulse to a value. This is the essence of initiative-taking people.

c) Initiative-taking People are driven by values – carefully thought about, selected and Internalized. They are still influenced by things that happen outside themselves, but their response to these happening is a value-based choice or response.

The mirror image of responsibility is ownership. Responsibility and ownership are twin brothers.

d) Taking ownership means not to blame anybody else for things that go wrong, but to ensure that something is done proactively.

e) Responsibility means being accountable, reliable, dependable, trustworthy, and taking control.

f) It implies that you will think before you act and that you will consider the possible consequences for all people affected by your actions.

g) It means not making excuses.

h) It means not blaming others for your mistakes or taking credit for other's achievements. In this sense responsibility is in line with the Golden Rule of doing unto others, as you want them to do unto you.

i) Responsibility means taking ownership of your behaviour and living with the consequences of your behaviour.

j) Taking responsibility means not doing things without thinking about the consequences of your actions.

k) With every right (provided by law) goes a responsibility. On their own, rights become dangerous.

l) Responsible behaviour involves a commitment to distinguish between right and wrong and to do the right thing.

m) Responsible behaviour involves sticking to good convictions and living out your values.

n) Involvement is a catchphrase for responsibility. The responsible person will be involved with the people around him.

o) Responsible means being dependable.

p) Responsible behaviour means to act like a "reasonable man" (legal term).

q) A value-based approach to life means that what I do must add value.

r) Being responsible means keeping in mind that you are responsible to a higher authority.

s) Being responsible also implies that you pursue excellence. You do your best with what you have. You keep trying and do not quit or give up easily.

t) Being responsible also means to exercise self-control and to be disciplined.

u) Being responsible also means not resisting actively or passively the explicit rules set out by the community. This would include following specified procedures even when not supervised or likely to be evaluated (e.g., the a student who keeps doing homework and study every day, even if he knows there will not be checking of books that day).

v) It means taking initiative to do those things that need to be done even when they are not specifically specified by the community's rules. This type of behavior is in keeping with the spirit of the rules: the performance beyond the call of duty.

w) The concept of Ubuntu implies that a person will be trustworthy. This is nothing else than being responsible.

When the group reports back on the question about responsible and irresponsible behaviour, divide the flip chart paper into two columns. On the left, write examples of responsible behaviour, and on the right, write examples of irresponsible behaviour. The following may come out otherwise; enrich the discussion with the following:

Responsible Behaviour	Irresponsible Behaviour
Stick to your good values	Unfaithfulness
to ensure that you do not get a NEGATIVE MINDSET	Being selfish
Develop your mindset into a positive mindset	Don't develop your mindset and be stuck to negative mindset
Look after your Spirit, mind and body health	Don't go to church, do not line up with ethics and neglect body health
Knowing your mindset status is a positive mindset.	Not being well-informed about NEGATIVE MINDSET
Not to lie about your status of mindset, but if you have negative space, seek help.	Not warning other people about the NEGATIVE MINDSET
Not to spread NEGATIVE MINDSET	Lying about your status of mindset

ITEM 6-4: THE FISH AND THE LOG

(5 Minutes)

Right down in big letters on a flip chart
"Will you be a fish or a log (a piece of wood)?"

Ask the group: What is the difference between how a river or stream affects a fish and a log? How can this be applied to our own lives in terms of taking responsibility?

Use the following ideas to help guide the feedback from the groups:

You can live your life like a fish or a log. Fish that live in rivers can swim upstream or with the current. If they stop swimming, they begin to float downstream. But by swimming upstream, fish can counter the natural flow of the stream and take advantage of what the river brings them. In contrast, logs just float. They have no choice but to go wherever the river takes them. The question for you now is, will you be part of the design of your future, or will you float into your future like a log in the river.

Taking responsibility for your life starts with a decision to become responsible. But it doesn't end with this decision. It is a lifelong process in which people realize things that are within their power and assume ownership of them. Responsible people take charge of themselves and their behaviour.

Assuming responsibility can be hard work, but the alternative is to stay dependent (something which may be easier but which leaves your life in the control of other people.)

By accepting responsibility for yourself and your behaviour, you will be able to live more like a fish than a log. You will make choices, pursue dreams and create opportunities for yourself rather than always having others decide these things for you.

BREAK

(5 Minutes)

ITEM 6-5: WHAT IS OUR RESPONSIBILITY TOWARDS THE NEGATIVE MINDSET PANDEMIC? (Exercise: 13)
In our Country, Society, Community, family, and individually

(30 Minutes)

Divide the participants in three groups: Let the participants in each group discuss one of the-following questions for 10 minutes. Let them give feedback afterwards for 5 minutes each.

a) Is there a connection between the spread of NEGATIVE MINDSET and irresponsibility?

b) What is required from us if we do not want to contribute to the spread of NEGATIVE MINDSET?

c) What does your religion teach you about responsible behaviour?

Use the following ideas to help guide the feedback from the groups:

The whole society is threatened by the threat of NEGATIVE MINDSET. The situation requires that everyone play a part in seeing to it that the virus does not spread further. Being personally responsible in regard to this pandemic would involve:

a) Abiding by behaviour that will eliminate the risk of spreading of NEGATIVE MINDSET, even when it might be possible to do irresponsible behaviour, without being caught out.

b) Making the internal decision not to be part of risk-taking behaviour, even if the temptation is tremendous.

Taking responsibility in a relationship implies taking responsibility for:

a) Your own health.

b) The other person's total well-being (Golden rule)

   i. The other person's health.

ii.   Guilty feelings

iii.   Relationship with God.

iv.   Relationship with parents.

c)   The consequences of your actions for third parties.

i.   Possible pregnancy and the impact on you as a couple.

ii.   The consequences of total responsibility for parenting for a possible baby.

d)   The consequence for the society's well-being.

i.   Do my actions contribute to immorality and licentiousness?

ii.   Do my actions/values contribute to the spread of NEGATIVE MINDSET?

Item 11-6: PERSONAL ACTION PLAN

(3 Minutes)

Write on your personal commitment sheet what you intend to do to increase your level of acting responsibly in future?

Will you walk the talk?

ITEM 11-7: CONCLUSION

(3 Minutes)

Remember the difference between a fish and a log. Remember the value framework that you identified at the beginning of this course and wrote on the personal commitment sheet that you are committed to. Is responsibility an integral part of that value framework? If it is, say to yourself: "Because I believe what I believe, I want to act responsibly." Then take responsibility for your life and choose your own destination.

In the next session we will go further with the theme of values. We are going to discuss that a responsible person is a person who holds the value of being fair, especially in the fight against NEGATIVE MINDSETS.

Session 12: Fairness

AIM. OBJECTIVES AND OUTLINE

Note to Facilitator. In the previous session we discussed the importance of being responsible in the fight against NEGATIVE MINDSET. The next session tries to convince participants that it is irresponsible and not fair to themselves and their loved ones to contract a NEGATIVE MINDSET and that it is also not fair to spread a NEGATIVE MINDSET. The participants are made aware of the fact that gender domination, as well as being prejudiced towards NEGATIVE MINDSET people, are ways of unfairness, contributing to the spread of NEGATIVE MINDSET. The conclusion must be to adhere to the Golden Rule, namely: Do unto others as you would like to be done unto.

Session Aim. By the end of this session, participants will appreciate the importance of the value of fairness in the prevention of the spread of NEGATIVE MINDSET.

Session Objectives. By the end of this session, participants will be able to:
   a) Describe fairness.
   b) Describe how fairness and unfairness are revealed in behaviour.
   c) Describe the practical implications of the value of fairness for sexual relationships.
   d) Recognize unfair practices in the handling of the NEGATIVE MINDSET pandemic.
   e) Recognize unfair practices due to gender inequality.

f) Understand the implications of the golden rule for everyday life.

g) Describe the relationship between the value of fairness and abstinence before marriage/faithfulness in marriage.

h) Know the dangers of unfairness in the spread of NEGATIVE MINDSET.

Session Outline

Introduction	5 minutes
Unpacking Fairness	30 minutes
Situations depicting unfairness or fairness	20 minutes
Ethical Frameworks and Fairness	25 minutes
Break	10 minutes
Role Play on Gender Equality	20 minutes
Group Discussion Gender Equality	60 minutes
Personal Action Plan	5 minutes
Conclusion	3 minutes
Total Time	178 minutes

PREPARATION

Preparation by Facilitator
None

Preparation by Participants
None

MATERIALS AND EQUIPMENT
Two slips with debate topic: Loyalty vs. Fairness

ITEM 7-1: UNPACKING FAIRNESS (Exercise: 14)

(30 Minutes)

Divide the participants in four groups. Request each group to discuss one of the following questions. Discuss for 10 minutes and give feedback for twenty minutes. Summarize at the end.

What do you understand about the term "Being fair"?

    a) What does it mean to be fair towards yourself in terms of sexuality?

    b) What does it mean to be fair towards the other person, when going into a sexual relationship with such a person?

    c) What does it mean to be fair toward third parties and the community when going into a sexual relationship with a person?

Use the following ideas to help guide the feedback from the groups:

a) Being Fair Implies

    i. Executing the Golden Rule: Do unto others as you want to be done unto.

    ii. Not taking away the ability of another person to make his/her own choices.

    iii. Being open-minded. Listen to others and try to understand what they are saying and feeling.

    iv. Making decisions that affect others only on appropriate considerations.

    v. Giving somebody an equal chance to" live, to grow, and to realize their potential.

b) Being fair towards yourself in terms of sexuality means:

    i. Do not induce guilty feelings in yourself just because of a lack of self-control.

    ii. If your parent's values are important for you, do not

reject their education and values just for the sake of desire.

c) Being fair towards the other person in terms of sexuality, means taking into consideration the Golden Rule in terms of:

    i.   That person's values, e.g., a commitment to virginity.

    ii.   That person's future, e.g., possible pregnancy vs. academic aspirations and financial security.

    iii.   That person's future dreams vs. being a NEGATIVE MINDSET.

    iv.   That person's love and commitment to his/her parents, as well as commitment to their expectations in terms of sexuality.

d) Being fair towards the community means:

    i.   Not contributing to the spirit of immorality and licentiousness.

    ii.   Not contributing to the spread of NEGATIVE MINDSET.

    iii.   Not contribute to placing a burden of orphans on the community.

    iv.   Not contributing to poverty by increasing medical costs, bail, teen pregnancies, and failing at school due to NEGATIVE MINDSET infection.

ITEM 7-2: SITUATIONS DEPICTING UNFAIRNESS OR FAIRNESS (Exercise 15)

(20 Minutes)

Divide the participants into five groups. Ask them to discuss whether there is unfairness (or fairness) in the following situations? Discuss 5 minutes and give feedback for 10 minutes.

- A person is married in a polygamous marriage but is not faithful to his/her partner(s).

- An unmarried person lies to his newly engaged partner, saying that he has never had sex before.
- An infected person, not knowing his status, who is sexually active.
- Old fling asking a student lover to leave school and be pregnant with his baby.
- Prejudice towards NEGATIVE MINDSET people.

ITEM 12-3: ETHICAL FRAME-WORK AND FAIRNESS (Exercise 16)

(25 Minutes)

Ask the participants to form three groups. Let each group discuss one of the following questions for five minutes. Give feedback afterward.

a) What is your religion's View on fairness in everyday life?
b) How does the philosophy of Ubuntu relate to "being fair"?
c) What do you think will be difficult when you apply fairness in all your relationships?

(10 Minutes)

ITEM 12-4: ROLE-PLAY ON GENDER EQUALITY (EXERCISE 17)

(20 Minutes)

Divide the participants into two groups. Let each group do one of the following role-plays. Give them ten minutes to prepare and five minutes to present. Afterwards, let them point out the unfairness in terms of gender equality and ask them what makes it difficult to apply fairness in these circumstances.

a) <u>Group 1</u>. A rural man who believes in polygamy comes home and tells his wife that he is going to marry a second wife. The wife is totally against this second marriage. She tells him about the dangers of NEGATIVE MINDSET and that she feels rejected. The husband just ignores her opposition.

b) <u>Group 2.</u> A woman who suffered from depression went to a psychologist. He informed her that because both she and her husband are working, she must negotiate with him that they equally take responsibility for work in the house, e.g. cooking and washing dishes. The man refuses and tells her it is not a man's job. When she continues with her argument, he assaults her.

ITEM 12-5: GROUP DISCUSSION ON GENDER EQUALITY (Exercise 18)

Divide the participants into four groups. Let each group discuss the following questions for 30 minutes and thereafter give feedback for 30 minutes.

<u>Group 1: The Role and Nature of Men and Women</u>
a) Are the differences between men and women only physiological, or do they differ fundamentally in their innermost nature?
b) What implications do these have for the roles of men and women in society?
c) What is your religion's view on the roles of men and women?
d) What implications are the above for NEGATIVE MINDSET prevention?

<u>Group 2: Gender Domination</u>
a) Why is gender equality important in the fight against NEGATIVE MINDSET prevention?
b) Does submissiveness still have a place in society?

c) What are the dangers of gender domination?

d) What implications do the above have for NEGATIVE MINDSET prevention?

Group 3: Negative Behavior

a) What would the implications of Ubuntu be for gender domination, e.g., valuing the good of the community above self-interest and showing respect to others?

b) How would the application of sound values change the stereotypes and the roles of men and women?

c) Is there an unbalanced viewpoint pressing for gender equality? What would be a balanced viewpoint?

Group 4: Values and Gender Equality

a) What are the implications of the six values that we have discussed, namely love, responsibility, integrity, fairness, respect, and professionalism for gender equality?

Use the following ideas to help guide the feedback from the groups:
It is well accepted that gender inequality in South Africa, especially in rural areas, contributes much to the rapid spread of NEGATIVE MINDSET. How very, gender inequality is not restricted to rural areas but appears in all spheres of life. Problems with gender equality are a manifestation of a lack of application of values, especially lack of respect and lack of fairness. It is therefore not in line with the Golden Rule.

ITEM 12-6: PERSONAL ACTION PLAN

(13 Minutes)

Write in the space next to question 6 on your personal commitment sheet what you intend to do in the future to increase your level of acting fairly?

Will you walk the talk?

ITEM 12-7: CONCLUSION

(13 Minutes)

If I choose a value framework in which fairness is an integral part and live up to my value system, I will contribute to the fight against NEGATIVE MINDSET. Then, my point of departure will be: "Because I believe what I believe, I will act in fairness to everybody around me. This will include sexuality. I do it, because I have committed myself to the Golden Rule of doing unto others as I want them to do unto me."

In the next session we will discover that if you want to call yourself a person with integrity, you need to be trustworthy.

Session 13: Integrity

AIM, OBJECTIVES, AND OUTLINE

Note to Facilitator. The seventh session addresses the value of integrity. A person with integrity is a person who is loyal towards other people and can be trusted. If we act with integrity, we will act with caring love; we will act responsibly and with fairness towards other people. That means that we will be true to all our promises and that we will not be unfaithful in our relationships. In the life of a person with integrity, dishonesty and extramarital relationships do not have a place; trust will never be betrayed. I will act in line with the Golden Rule. What I do in the dark, I must be able to defend in the light.

Session Aim. By the end of this session, participants will be able to define integrity, trust, and loyalty.

Session Objectives
By the end of this session, participants will be able to:
   a) Describe the importance of integrity.
   b) Realize that it includes trust and loyalty.
   c) Describe ways/methods of implementing integrity, trust, and loyalty.
   d) Describe the influence of the lack of integrity on the spread of NEGATIVE MINDSET.

Session Outline

Unpacking Integrity	20 minutes
Video: Loyalty	40 minutes
Integrity and Sexuality	25 minutes
Personal Action Plan	3 minutes
Conclusion	3 minutes
Total Time	91 minutes

PREPARATION

Preparation by Facilitator
None

Preparation by Participant
None

MATERIALS AND EQUIPMENT

ITEM 8-1: UNPACKING INTEGRITY (Exercise 19)

(20 Minutes)

Announce the theme. Tell the participants that Integrity also includes trust and loyalty. Divide into three groups and let each group discuss for 8 minutes one of the following topics. Thereafter let them give feedback for 12 minutes.

a) Group 1: What do you understand about the term "Integrity"?

b) Group 2: What do you understand under the term "Trust"?

c) Group 3: What do you understand under the term "Loyalty"?

Use the following ideas to help guide the feedback from the groups on Integrity:

Make them aware that integrity, to a great extent, includes trust and loyalty.

Integrity means to be reliable.

Integrity means to stand up for your beliefs about right and wrong.

It means to be your best self, and to resist social pressures to do things you know are wrong.

Integrity is being able to defend and not being ashamed of what you do when nobody can see you.

It is to walk the talk.

It is keeping your word, honouring your commitments, paying your debts, and returning what you have borrowed.

Integrity means to be honest and trustworthy, which is in line with the concept of Ubuntu.

Integrity means acting in line with the Golden Rule of doing unto others as you do.

Would like them to do unto you.

Integrity is a *principle* of viewing yourself as a person with integrity, and acting in such a way that other people also view you as a person with integrity.

Integrity goes with character building.

It takes years to build your name but moments to throw it away.

What *I* do *in* the dark, I must be able to defend in the day (comment: *Something* that *is* not *possible if* you have a "kelpie". Umshimbilili)

The following are also characteristics of trust and loyalty.

Loyalty means:
- To stand by, support, and protect your family, friends,

employers, community, and country.
- Not belittling or talking negatively.
- Not talking behind people's backs.
- To be open without secrets.
- Dependable and reliable.
- Causing no undue hurt or discomfort that you would not want done unto you.
- Being around when needed.
- Not misusing, abusing, or stealing.
- Not dealing with untruths.
- Not deceiving, misleading, or being devious and tricky.
- Not betraying trust.
- Not withholding important information in relationships of trust.
- Telling the truth even if it hurts.

Trust means:
- Being sincere.
- Honouring obligations.
- Being fair in dealings – not taking sides.
- Making partner/organization a high priority.
- Sacrificing for the other. (Unselfish)

Trust is built when people recognize that you act in line with the Golden Rule of doing unto others as you want them to do unto you.

Misplaced trust is one of the major causes of NEGATIVE MINDSET. Many spouses have been infected due to trust in an unfaithful partner. Trustworthy partners, on the other hand, are the best security against NEGATIVE MINDSET.

ITEM 13-5
A role-play can be done on a person who is confronted by a

friend about his disloyalty in his marriage. The friend may, in his confrontation, first make.

As if it is the behavior of another person. Then, like Nathan in the Bible, with King David, he may say: "It is you, acting unfaithful to your marriage partner".

Afterwards have a discussion and list which values a person with an extramarital affair negates. What is the influence of such relationships on the spread of NEGATIVE MINDSET? Stress again that a person with an extramarital affair does not act in line with the Golden Rule.

ITEM 8-3: INTEGRITY AND SEXUALITY (Exercise: 20)

(25 Minutes)

Discuss the following in three groups for 10 minutes. Give feedback for 5 minutes per group. Summarize.

    a) What place does a condom have in the lives of people who have committed themselves to religious values and lifestyle if they see themselves as people with integrity, trust and loyalty?

    b) What is your religion's view on integrity?

    c) What makes it difficult to act according to the values of integrity, trust, and loyalty under all circumstances?

The following can be used to guide the discussion on condoms: even in marriage!

The effectiveness of condoms in protecting against NEGATIVE MINDSET and other sexually transmitted infections is a scientific rather than a moral issue. All the scientific evidence points in the same direction: correct and consistent use of condoms of good quality vastly reduces the likelihood of NEGATIVE MINDSET transmission. Among discordant couples (couples where just one partner is infected), those who always use condoms for sex have little or no risk of the virus passing to the uninfected partner, compared with couples who use condoms sporadically or not at all.

Remember that you are responsible for your own sexual health. The question is how much you want to rely on trust and integrity. Many people have the standpoint: "I do not rely on trust or on how healthy the person looks. I don't wait for the person to tell me if he/she is HIV positive or not. If I am willing to be sexually active, I am the only person to look after my health. Therefore, it is my responsibility, and not my partner's, to use a condom, whenever I have sex."

From my own side, however, if I see myself as a person with firm values, I must make a commitment to say that I am a person with integrity. I am trustworthy and loyal to my lifelong partner, and therefore, my lifelong partner will never have to fear infection coming from my side.

Condomizing can only play a role in a value-based relationship if it goes together with integrity. The true way of protecting yourself from distractions of life, like teen pregnancy, STD and HIV, is to abstain from Sex.

ITEM 8-4: PERSONAL ACTION PLAN

(3 Minutes)

Write in the space provided in question 7 on your personal commitment sheet what you intend to do to increase your level of acting with integrity, trustworthiness and loyalty in future?

ITEM 8-5: CONCLUSION

(3 Minutes)

In this session, we discovered that integrity is the characteristic that makes a person trustworthy. A person who sees himself as a person with integrity will never indulge In being unfaithful in relationships but will always be loyal. Such a person will also never contribute to the spread of a NEGATIVE MINDSET. Integrity flows from a strong commitment to a value framework: "Because I believe what I believe, I will always act with integrity, trustworthiness and loyalty."

In the next session we will see that a person with integrity is a person that will never takes advantage of another person but will respect others with the same respect that he/she has for him/herself.

Session 14: Respect

AIM, OBJECTIVES, AND OUTLINE

Note to Facilitator. This session addresses the value of respect. A person with integrity is a person who respects life, himself, and others. Respect for others means to acknowledge the worth of other people and that other people have the right to be free individuals. Respect, therefore, means that we will acknowledge the boundaries which others set for their interaction with us. This implies that I will not manipulate, exploit or take advantage of others or misuse them for personal gain or pleasure. This value correlates with the African value of "Ubuntu: I am because you are." It also correlates with the Golden Rule of doing unto others, as you want them to do unto you.

Session Aim. By the end of this session, participants will be able to recognize their own boundaries and will be able to treat others and themselves with respect.

Session Objectives. By the end of this session, participants will be able to:
   a) Describe what respect implies.
   b) Describe how respect can be applied in everyday life.
   c) Discuss the relationship between respect and boundaries.
   d) Understand the relationship between Ubuntu and NEGATIVE MINDSET.

Session Outline

Boundary Exercise	20 minutes
Unpacking Respect	30 minutes
Respect and Intimate Relationships	25 minutes
Ubuntu and the Fight Against NEGATIVE MINDSET-infection	20 minutes
Personal Action Plan	3 minutes
Conclusion	1 minute
Total Time	99 minutes

ITEM 9-1: BOUNDARY EXERCISE

(20 Minutes)

Let every participant pair up with another participant of the same gender. Give them the instructions and let them be in each position for about 45 seconds.

Find your partner now and wait for further directions.

a) First, stand as close or as far away from each other as you normally would to have a conversation. Tell one another about the pets you own or hobbies you have or sport you enjoy.

b) Now, I want you to stand back-to-back and discuss your favourite food.

c) Next, I want one of you to remain standing, while the other gets down on your knees. Talk about your favorite movie or book or song. (After a minute, tell the pairs to switch positions.)

d) Finally, I would like you to stand toe to toe and share the qualities you would like to see in the person you marry.

Ask the group:

a) In which position were you the most comfortable? Which was the most uncomfortable? Why?

b) Are there other boundaries, except for physical space, that people have that must be respected?

Use the following ideas to help guide the feedback from the groups

Perhaps you have one friend that likes to be hugged and one that doesn't. These, and what you experienced above, are examples of physical boundaries. We need to acknowledge our own boundaries and respect the boundaries of others.

We have many other kinds of social boundaries besides physical distance. We may have speech boundaries (things we dislike people saying to us), group boundaries (how many people we want to be with for how long a time), possession boundaries (what we are comfortable sharing or lending), etc.

In all these types of boundaries, there is the possibility of boundaries that are too rigid or too weak. Either one can lead to problems in relationships.

On the other hand, it is very important that we are sensitive towards these boundaries of other people and respect them. The quality of respect is related to the concept of boundaries. Because we respect others, and ourselves, we set boundaries that define who we are and what we value. With the help of healthy boundaries, we can define how we will react and behave in certain circumstances. This keeps us from acting impulsively on the whims of our desires or from being pressured by someone in the heat of the moment. Boundaries are an outgrowth of our respect for others and ourselves.

A very important way in which we show respect is the way we show respect to other people's boundaries. Every country in the world must establish and maintain clear boundaries between it and the surrounding countries. Often boundary disputes are a cause of conflict and even wars between countries.

In the same way, clear boundaries are important in all human relationships. Two rules about respect apply here: 1) Respect the boundaries of others, and 2) take responsibility for what is inside your boundaries. If you have healthy boundaries, you know who you are, and you have respect for the boundaries of others.

Respecting another person's boundaries is in line with the Golden Rule of doing unto others as you want them to do unto you.

ITEM 9-2: UNPACKING RESPECT (Exercise 21)

(30 Minutes)

Divide the participants into three groups. Ask every group to discuss two of the following questions for 10 minutes. Let them give feedback for 20 minutes. Summarize.

a) What do you understand under the term "Respect"?
b) What is self-respect?
c) How do I get others to respect me?
d) What type of behaviour reveals that you do not have respect as a personal value?
e) What is the relationship between respect for life and NEGATIVE MINDSET prevention?
f) What are your religions' views on respect?

Use the following ideas to help guide the feedback from the groups:

Definition of Respect

Respect can be defined as an acknowledgement of the worth of another person and his/her right as a free individual. Respect is revealed in unconditional care for and warmth towards another person and in the quality of attention that is given to another person.

Respect Also Means

- To be courteous and polite.
- To judge all people on their merits.
- To be tolerant, appreciative, and accepting of individual differences.
- To respect the right of individuals to make decisions about their own lives.
- Not to abuse, demean, or mistreat anyone.
- Not to use, manipulate, exploit, or take advantage of others.
- To see value and worth in people.
- To acknowledge the uniqueness of other people.
- To believe people have innate dignity and purpose. To respect personal autonomy.
- To respect privacy.
- To show hospitality.
- To show kindness, friendliness, and helpfulness. To treat other people well.
- To be fair, not taking sides.
- To show that you place a high value on another person by how you speak about or treat them or something that is an important part of their life.

- To show respect is to show that you appreciate and accept individual differences. Respect is courteous and polite. Respect never abuses, demeans, or mistreats. Respect would not take advantage of others or manipulate them and use them for personal gain or pleasure.

All these characteristics of respecting others is embedded in the concept of Ubuntu.

Self-respect Means

To show pride in oneself (Neatness, health consciousness, posture, communication). This normally reveals your mindset if you are a negative or a positive in mindset.

How do I get others to respect me?

Respect is earned by behaving responsibly and by respecting others. Acting irresponsible will not earn you respect.

ITEM 14-3: RESPECT AND INTIMATE RELATIONSHIPS (Exercise 22)

(25 Minutes)

Divide in two groups, preferably men in one group and ladies in the other group. Let both groups discuss all the following questions for 15 minutes. Give feedback for 10 minutes:

- a) What respect do women deserve in intimate relationships?
- b) What respect do men deserve in intimate relationships?
- c) What do you think will be the most difficult part when you apply respect in all aspects in your relationship with a permanent partner?

ITEM 9-4: UBUNTU AND THE FIGHT AGAINST NEGATIVE MINDSET-INFECTION

Discuss in groups for 10 minutes:

What can the value of Ubuntu contribute to the fight against NEGATIVE MINDSET?

Use the following ideas to help guide the feedback from the groups:

Ubuntu is a traditional African approach towards life's challenges. Ubuntu means to be human, respect the worth of the human being, value the good of the community above self-interest, strive to help other people in the spirit of service, show respect to others, and be honest and trustworthy. Ubuntu is therefore also in line with the Golden Rule of doing unto others as you want them to do unto you.

Ubuntu's emphasis on working together and respecting human dignity is a very important principle in the fight against NEGATIVE MINDSET. It emphasizes a collaborative spirit, promoting a shared will to survive.

ITEM 9-5: Personal Action Plan

Write on your personal commitment sheet what you intend to do to increase your level of acting with respect?

Will you walk the talk?

ITEM 14-6: Conclusion

Sum up by saying: When we started this course, you stated to which value-framework you are committed. Is respect part of that value framework? Then you can say: "Because I believe what I believe, I will treat others with respect. I will act in line with the Golden Rule and treat others with the respect that I want for myself." If we all respect other people, and ourselves,

NEGATIVE MINDSET will not spread.

In the next session we will talk about the value of professionalism. Respect for life, yourself and others is an integral part of professionalism.

Session 15: Professionalism

AIM, OBJECTIVES, AND OUTLINE

Note to Facilitator. A person acting professionally is a person who acts according to all the values that have already been discussed. In this session, we shortly integrate these different values, in the discussions. Not much new information will come out during these discussions.

Session Aim. By the end of this session, participants should be able to embrace professionalism as a personal value and seek to instil it into others to combat NEGATIVE MINDSET.

Session Objectives. By the end of this session, participants will be able to:

a) Describe which aspects of professionalism are relevant to NEGATIVE MINDSET.

b) Describe the impact of a professional attitude on the prevention of the spread of NEGATIVE MINDSET.

Session Outline

Unpacking professionalism and its possible relationship to NEGATIVE MINDSET prevention	20 minutes
Gatekeeper of Professionalism	20 minutes
Personal Action Plan	3 minutes
Conclusion	1 minute
Total Time	44 minutes

PREPARATION

Preparation by Facilitator
None

Preparation by Participants
None

ITEM 10-1: UNPACKING PROFESSIONALISM AND ITS POSSIBLE RELATIONSHIP TO NEGATIVE MINDSET-PREVENTION (Exercise 23)

(20 Minutes)

Divide the group in smaller groups. Let each group investigate how the following character traits of a person, whose behavior is professional, can contribute to the combat of the spread of NEGATIVE MINDSET.

    a) Leading by example with honourable behaviour
    b) Self-disciplined and Self-control
    c) Integrity and Honesty

Use the following idea to help guide the feedback:
People who act professionally in the fight against NEGATIVE MINDSET will:

a) Lead by example
    i. Know their own status of mindset.
    ii. Inspire others to know their status of mindset.
    iii. Live a life according to high ethical values.
    iv. Take the consequences of deeds into consideration before they decide on a deed.
    v. Take responsibility for the consequences of their deeds.
b) Act with self-discipline and self-control.
    i. Exercise self-control over their own urges.

ii.   Make conscious decisions about his health and success.

iii.   Not lead other into temptation of high-risk behavior.

c) Act with integrity and honesty.

    i.   Not make themselves guilty of unfaithfulness.

    ii.   Do not indulge in unscrupulous relationships.

    iii.   Not tolerate the ethical misbehaviour of another person.

ITEM 10-2: (OPTIONAL) GATEKEEPER OF PROFESSIONALISM (Exercise 24)

(120 Minutes)

Discuss the following scenario in two groups for 10 minutes, and give feedback for 10 minutes.

You are on a project, and you see that a married man is going on a date with a divorced woman to a movie, while his wife is under the impression that he is working late because he has a task to complete. What should be a professional response?

Use the following ideas to help guide the feedback from the group:

Part of professionalism is also to be the gatekeeper of professionalism.

Emphasize that the misbehaviour of any other person is also part of the business of the professional person.

A person has the right to mess up his own life, but they are not allowed to affect other's lives negatively.

ITEM 15-5: PERSONAL ACTION PLAN

(13 Minutes)

Write on YOUR personal commitment sheet what you intend to do to increase your level of acting with professionalism?

Will you walk the talk?

ITEM 10-6: Conclusion

A person acting professionally can contribute a lot to curb the spread of NEGATIVE MINDSET, by watching his own behavior as well as by being the gatekeeper of professionalism in other's lives.

We have now completed the module on the different values of love that care: responsibility, fairness, integrity, respect, and professionalism. We will now proceed to the module on skills necessary to live according to these values to combat NEGATIVE MINDSET. The first and probably the most important skill is the ability to make value-based decisions. This will be discussed in the next session.

Module IV

Skills Needed To Combat the Negative Mindset-Infection

Session 16: Making Positive Life-Style Choices

AIM, OBJECTIVES, AND OUTLINE

Note to Facilitator. In the previous session, we established which values are needed to combat NEGATIVE MINDSET. From this session onwards, the programme starts to address the skills needed to combat the possibility of NEGATIVE MINDSET. The first skill that the programme wants to teach participants is how to make positive lifestyle choices based on their values. The participant must be led into making decisions that are on the basis of caring love, responsibility, fairness towards others, respect for the boundaries of others, and exemplifying integrity, trust and loyalty.

Session Aim. By the end of this session, participants will be able to make positive value-based lifestyle choices that may protect them from becoming infected with the NEGATIVE MINDSET.

Session Objectives. By the end of this session, participants will be able to:
 a) Work through a systematic decision-making process in response to a given situation.
 b) Know what factors to take into consideration to make decisions that will lead to ethical conduct.
 c) Describe the value of listening to your conscience when making decisions.

Session Outline

Crossroads Metaphor: Deciding which way to go	15 minutes
The seven-step decision-making process	10 minutes
Practicing the seven steps	50 minutes
Your conscience and decisions	20 minutes
Personal Action Plan	3 minutes
Total Time	101 minutes

PREPARATION

Preparation by Facilitator
None

Preparation by Participants
None

MATERIALS AND EQUIPMENT
Flip chart and Koki's

ITEM 11-1: CROSSROADS METAPHOR: DECIDING WHICH WAY TO GO

(115 Minutes)

Draw a crossroads picture on a flipchart.

Tell the group **that** a person called Peter is driving in a car and wants to go to a holiday resort at the sea. Draw a little block, indicating where the car is currently. Tell them that as he is driving along the road, he reaches a crossroad. The driver does not know which way to go. He stops and switches off the car. Ask the group: What must happen for Peter to make a decision which way to go? Which steps can they identify?

Lead the group into answering the following:
Step 1. The driver must realize that he has a problem and that he needs to solve it. He wants to reach a certain destination, and if he does not make the right choices, he may never reach that destination. He must clarify precisely how big his problem is. The driver must read all the information, telling him which places the different roads lead. If the directions on the road signs are clear and give him enough direction, the problem is easily solved. If there are no road signs, his problem expands. He must, therefore, clarify his problem.

Step 2. Then, he must start gathering all the information that he needs. He must keep in mind:

i.   His own goal, namely the holiday resort.
ii.   The conditions of the roads – Are all of them tarred, or are there some gravel roads?
iii.   The direction in which he and his passengers think the holiday resort is situated.

Step 3. The driver should then make a list of his options. There are four roads in four directions. He has to take one of them.

Step 4. The driver should evaluate the options. He knows that he can't go back because the holiday resort is not behind him. Maybe the one road going straight on is a small bad gravel road, which looks as if it is very seldom used. So, he may decide to discard that option. So there are only two options left. Maybe he has an idea that the sea is not to his left, and therefore, keeping in mind that his goal is to go to the sea, he may decide not to take the road to the left.

Step 5. Now, the driver makes a decision about which option he will take, namely, to take the road to the right.

Step 6. He begins to act and implements his decision. He starts his car, puts it into gear, and turns off to the right.

ITEM 11-2: THE SEVEN-STEP DECISION MAKING PROCESS
(10 Minutes)

Making use of the metaphor of the crossroads informs the group that all wise decisions involve a six-step process. This process could lead to a healthier, more productive and satisfying life when faithfully applied. But, if you want to live a value-based lifestyle, there is one ultimate test that forms an extra step. Then it becomes a seven-step process. The seven steps are the following:

a) Clarify the problem. Whose problem is it? Who is the best one to solve it? What do I want to achieve? What is my goal or purpose?

b) What information and facts can I gather that will influence my decision?

c) Make a list of all your options. What are your alternative solutions to the problem? There are almost always more than two options, so if you are stuck, get help thinking of more alternatives.

d) Evaluate each of your options. Predict what the consequences might be of each of your options. Make sure your options

   i. Are legal.
   ii. Help achieve goals previously set.
   iii. Are in line with the authority in charge.
   iv. Treat others kindly
   v. Build relationships. 16-5

a) **Decide which option is best.** Make sure that your choice will support what is really important to you and will help you achieve your goals. Test your decision. Is it practical? Can it be carried out? Is it the best in the long term? How will the decision influence your situation today and affect your life tomorrow? Can you cope with the responsibilities and consequences of your decision?

b) **The ultimate test.**

    I.   Is this decision according to my values?

        1. What would my Creator say about this option?

        2. Would my Creator have chosen this option?

        3. Does my conscience give me total peace about this decision?

        4. Does my choice demonstrate love, responsibility, integrity, fairness, and respect?

        5. Is my decision in line with the Golden Rule of doing unto others as I want them to do unto me?

    II.   In the African context, the question can also be asked: Is this decision in the spirit of Ubuntu?

c) **Design a plan to carry out your decision.** After a decision is made, you have set or clarified a goal for yourself. This will now require some sort of action on your part. Advise the people who are affected by your decisions.

Ask the group if there is one of them that can repeat the seven steps without looking at the notes.

ITEM 11-3: PRACTICING THE SEVEN-STEP DECISION-MAKING PROCESS

(50 Minutes)

Divide the participants into four groups. Give each group one of the following problems. Plan for 10 minutes of discussion and then 10 minute of feedback for each group. Emphasize to them that they must clearly md1cate the seven steps on a flip chart in their feedback. Afterwards, they must answer the following questions:

d) What in your decisions reveals the values that you have in your life?

e) What are the important values that help you choose between the different options?

    I.   Group 1. You have *noticed* that your partner has been acting strangely over the past few weeks. You have the suspicion that he/she is unfaithful towards you. Use the seven-step decision-making process to come to a decision on a plan of action.

    II.   Group 2. You have discovered that you are infected with NEGATIVE MINDSET. You are married but have not been faithful to your wife. Now that you know that you are infected, what are you *going* to do? Use the seven-step decision-making process to come to a decision on a plan of action.

    III.   Group 3. You are a 20-year-old person. You must make a decision about sexuality for the rest of your life. Are you choosing permanent celibacy, abstinence till marriage, or condomizing? Use the seven-step decision-making process to come to a decision on this issue.

    IV.   Group 4. You are a young person who has moved out of your parent's home recently. You must make a decision about your religious involvement for the rest of your life. Are you choosing to be dedicated and involved in activities, *dedicated* but not involved, or are you going to let religion have a low profile in your life? Use the seven-step decision-making process to come to a decision on this issue.

Use the following ideas to help guide the feedback from the groups:

Remember, there are no absolute correct/right answers in these scenarios. The important things are:

a) Following the different steps in the process.

b) Considering your values.

We must understand that mature decision-making also includes the following:

a) Not being unduly influenced by our emotions.
b) Knowing our value system.
c) Taking responsibility for our decisions.

Always remember that a human is someone who can make his own choices. If you go out with your date tonight, you have a choice. You are in control. You can decide for yourself: Who am I taking out? Where are we going? What are we going to do? How far are we going to go in our physical relationship?

When do I want to have sex?

That is human – you have a choice – you are in control. An animal has no choice. You know what happens when a dog in the street is in heat – all the male dogs in the neighbourhood would mill around that house. They may even jump the fence just to reach the female that is in heat. They are driven by their passion. They have no control, and they take no responsibility for what they do. They have only one thing on their minds: to satisfy their own sexual desire.

ITEM 11-4: YOUR CONSCIENCE AND DECISIONS (Exercise 25)
(20 Minutes)

Discuss the following questions:

a) What is your conscience?
b) What is the relationship between your conscience and your values?
c) What role does your conscience play when you make decisions?
d) How can you sharpen your conscience and your ability to listen to your conscience?
e) What makes it difficult to listen to your conscience when making decisions in everyday life?

Use the following ideas to help guide the feedback from the groups:

Your conscience is formed by all your experiences and is, in a certain sense, a summary of your values and value framework. It is used by the mind to guide behaviour. You can make the decision whether you want to listen to your conscience or not.

ITEM 11-5: PERSONAL ACTION PLAN

Write on your personal commitment sheet what you intend to do in future to increase your level of making positive value-based decisions.

Will you walk the talk?

ITEM 11-6: CONCLUSION

(3 Minutes)

Remind the group of the values of love, responsibility, fairness, integrity and respect, which flow from a commitment to a higher-order commitment to a value framework. Tell them to always remember that they do not just make decisions if they want to make good decisions. It is "Because I believe what I believe, that I want to make good value-based decisions." Remind them of the most important of the seven steps and urge them to follow them in all decisions they make.

Inform them that in the next session we are going to deal with the skill of assertiveness which is necessary in order to stick to value-based decisions.

Session 17: Defending Your Decisions (Assertiveness)

AIM, OBJECTIVES, AND OUTLINE

Note to Facilitator. In the previous session, we handled the skill of value-based decision-making. In this session, the programme wants to empower the individual to be able to live according to his values and decisions without being sidetracked by peer pressure or by dominating people. The session wants to teach participants how to act assertively and how to communicate their viewpoints in such a way that what they say is not easily ignored. It is done by contrasting assertive communication with passive and aggressive communication of your views.

Session Aim. By the end of this session, participants will have discovered how to apply the skill of being assertive.

Session Objectives. By the end of this session, participants will be able to:
a) Utilize strategies to assertively communicate their decisions.
b) Have specific responses to give to someone who won't take "no" for an answer the first time.

Session Outline

What is Assertiveness?	5 minutes
What is the recipe to act assertively?	5 minutes
Practicing the three steps of assertiveness	25 minutes
Break	5minutes
The influence of self-esteem on vulnerability to NEGATIVE MINDSET-infection	25 minutes
Improving your self-esteem	10 minutes
Religion and Assertiveness	20minutes
Personal Action Plan	3 minutes
Conclusion	3 minutes
Total Time	131 minutes

PREPARATION

Preparation by Facilitator

None

Preparation by Participants

None

MATERIALS AND EQUIPMENT

Slide on the definition of assertiveness.

ITEM 12-1: WHAT IS ASSERTIVENESS?

(5 Minutes)

Emphasize that this is one of the most important skills that a person needs to live a value-based life, as well as not become a NEGATIVE MINDSET

Ask the group what assertiveness is. When they give feedback,

use a slide or transparency with the following:
a) To stand up for your rights without intruding on the rights of others.
b) It is the other side of the Golden Rule: Do unto yourself as you would like them to do unto you.
c) Being confident but not demanding.
d) Expressing negative and positive feelings.
e) To express yourself honestly, without distortion, without exaggeration, and without putting yourself in the foreground.
f) In Afrikaans the term means "Selfhandhawing", or "Selfgeldend".

Use the following ideas to help guide the participants to understand assertiveness:

a) By standing up for my rights, I respect myself and will receive it from others.
b) By trying to never hurt anybody, in the end, I do hurt other people, including myself.
c) By sacrificing your own rights, relationships are sometimes broken, and others are prevented from developing.
d) It is a form of selfishness to keep my thoughts and feelings to myself.
e) Sacrificing my rights teaches others to disregard me.
f) If I do not let other people know how their behavior affects me negatively; I deprive them of the opportunity to change their behavior.
g) I can decide what is important to me. It is not necessary to live under the tyranny of "must'.
h) I feel better about myself if I do what I believe is right for me. This makes my relationships with others

satisfactory.

i) I can expect other's courteousness and respect.

j) I have the right to express myself as I would like to because I do not want to get a NEGATIVE MINDSET.

k) In assertiveness, we can distinguish between conviction and preference. "Is this choice of mine only a preference, or is it a conviction for which I will stand, even if I must die for it?"

l) When, in my decisions, it goes about values, then it is about convictions. I will stand by my convictions, because it bears witness of my integrity. I will not bow from the values of love, responsibility, fairness, integrity and respect.

ITEM 12-3: WHAT 15 THE RECIPE TO BE ABLE TO ACT ASSERTIVELY?

(5 Minutes)

Ask the participants to identify steps that will assist them in acting more assertively in most situations.

Enrich with: The important three steps are

a) Step 1. Acknowledge the other person's feelings, that he may feel bad about your perspective.

b) Step 2. Give your perspective/request clearly.

c) Step 3. Give your reasons.

Examples:

"I know that you are going to feel hurt/ unhappy if I say this to you, but No. The reason is that I."

"I know that you may feel that we are too busy this afternoon, but I would like to ask to take off this afternoon. The reason is

"Good advice when you want to say "NO!" Always say it early on.

Have an alternative solution: "No, but what about..."

ITEM 12-4: PRACTICING THE THREE STEPS OF ASSERTIVENESS (Exercise 26)

(25 Minutes)

Divide into three groups. Let each group role play a specific situation. Let the one person react with the three steps of assertiveness against the w/11 of the other person. Emphasize that the three steps must be clearly visible during the relationship.

a) A man and a man, both married and working together, start to feel attracted to each other. One tries to go further with the relationship, and the other one declines.

b) An unmarried man tries to convince his girlfriend that it is OK to have sex if they use a condom, while she feels that it is against her values. Let this group do this role-play three times, first acting in a non-assertive way, then in an assertive way and then in an aggressive way.

c) An unmarried instructor declines an invitation to have sex with a female student in exchange for an exam paper.

After the role-plays, ask the group to reflect on their experience of the role-play. Use the following to guide the feedback.

There is enormous pressure on young people to become sexually active. The media are telling you to go for it. Your friends talk as if it is so uncool not to be sexually active. You sound as if you are the odd one out. Your boyfriend says: "Trust me" or "If you really love me... "Be honest with him. Tell him if he really loves you, he will exchange it for love.

Remember the following response, which a girl gave to her friends when her friends were putting pressure on her to become sexually active. She said: "Remember, I could become like any of you within five minutes, but not one of you can become like me again!"

BREAK

(5 Minutes)

ITEM 12-5: THE INFLUENCE OF SELF-ESTEEM ON VULNERABILITY TO NEGATIVE MINDSET- INFECTION (Exercise 27)

(25 Minutes)

Keep the participants in the same groups and discuss the following questions:
   a)   What is the influence of your self-esteem?
   b)   The quality of choices you make?
   c)   Acting assertively and living according to your values?
   d)   Your vulnerability to NEGATIVE MINDSET infection?

Use the following ideas to help guide the feedback from the groups:
a)   Our self-esteem has to do with:
   i.   A feeling of being accepted. This is a feeling that we are valued for who we are and not for what we do or what we have. Every person wants to feel that you belong. If a person should feel that he belongs nowhere, then he feels lonely. This feeling of loneliness lowers a person's self-esteem.
   ii.   A feeling of own worth. This has to do with our relationship with ourselves.
   iii.   A feeling of competency. This is a feeling that a person is able to handle all situations. The feeling of being competent is the basic feeling underlying self-

confidence.

a) Your self-esteem develops as a result of your interactions with other people. It happens when we interact with other people. The result of these interactions forms our self-concept. Every day, we receive slaps on the back or slaps in the face. These reactions of other people influence our self-concept. How you incorporate these experiences in your life determines your self-concept. If you have low self-esteem, you will expect failures to happen to you. All expectations in connection with future events will be seen through the spectacles of the failures of the past, in the spirit of Ubuntu, where I value the good of the community above self-interest and of the Golden. Rule means that I will never contribute to breaking down the self-esteem of others.

b) The characteristics of a person with a positive self-image are the following:

    i. A person with a good self-image will not brag but is also not ashamed of talking about himself.

    ii. A person with a good self-image focuses just as much on other people as on him/herself. He is interested in other people.

    iii. He accepts others as they are and does not want to change them.

    iv. He can accept criticism and handle it constructively.

    v. He does not have the need to prove himself to others. He feels at ease in the company of others. This last characteristic is a very important one as this decreases such a person's vulnerability.

The person who has a low sense of self-worth has nothing about himself or herself to protect. So there is no reason to postpone pleasure, avoid dangerous behaviours, be concerned about the future, invest in education or health, or try to change the things about life that are wrong and unjust.

The person with a high sense of self-worth is motivated by the promise of the greater good to postpone immediate gratification of impulses. He or she has reasons to avoid dangerous behaviours that include an investment in the future, education and health. He knows he wants the best because he is worth the best. She knows she is worth waiting for because she is a quality person.

People with high self-esteem feel confident enough to make decisions based on their values. They turn down options which are not in line with their values.

ITEM 12-6: IMPROVING YOUR SELF-ESTEEM?

(10 Minutes)

Ask the groups to discuss the following question: "How can you improve your self-esteem?" and give feedback.
Use the following ideas to help guide the feedback from the groups:

a) Positive self-talk. A person's whole life can be determined by the way a person has become accustomed to talking to himself about himself. Some people are accustomed to always talking negatively towards themselves. They talk themselves down until nothing is left of their self-image and self-worth. When their team is playing a game, they. Prepare themselves that the team is going to lose, even if the team is ahead in the score. When they plan a project, they tell themselves that the project is going to fail. When they come home after a day's work, they only tell their spouse about everything that went wrong that day. They fill their minds so much with negative things about themselves and their surroundings that there Is nothing in their experience of life that makes it worth going on.

b) Positive talk to others. It is not only your self-talk that counts. Learn to talk to others in a positive tone. Focus on your successes and the things that you have achieved when you talk to other people. This does not mean that you must boast. It means that when you had a good day at work, and you see a friend after the day's work, you will say: "I had a very good day; I got a lot of work done, and I feel good about it." It is a very positive way of programming yourself and helps others to see you in a positive light.

c) Create a positive physical image of yourself. We do not always realize that the way we stand, sit or walk influences others' view of us. Their response to these may have an influence on our self-image.

d) Positive behaviour. If you act in an irresponsible manner, e.g. if you do not keep appointments, if you do not care for yourself, or if you do not pay your accounts, you will never develop a positive sense of identity. In other words, if you do not act according to the Golden Rule, you will not develop a positive sense of identity.

e) Take care of yourself. A sense of identity begins with taking care of yourself. You need to provide for your bodily needs (food, warmth, and shelter), keep your house clean, take care of your body, and eat correctly. Your needs for physical safety can be met by living in a place where people do not abuse you. You can develop emotional security to prevent your life from being only a series of changes.

ITEM 12-7: RELIGION AND ASSERTIVENESS (Exercise 28)

(20 Minutes)

Discuss in groups and give feedback:

a)   What does my religion say about assertiveness?
b)   What does my religion say about positive self-esteem?
c)   What do you think will be very difficult when you apply assertiveness in your relationships?

ITEM 12-8: PERSONAL ACTION PLAN

Write on your personal commitment sheet what you intend to do in future to increase your level of acting with assertiveness.
Will you walk the talk?

ITEM 12-9: CONCLUSION

(3 Minutes)

Assertive behaviour is very important if you want to stick to your convictions and your values. It helps you to act with integrity. Therefore, you can say, "Because I believe what I believe, I will act with integrity."

Assertive behaviour is normal. By expressing your wishes openly and with self-confidence, you give others the liberty to do the same. It is, therefore, totally in line with the Golden Rule. However, it is necessary to do it tactfully and to listen to the other person.

If you know how to act assertively, the risk of getting a NEGATIVE MINDSET will decline; for that, you have to work on developing positive self-esteem. The temptation of high- risk sexual behaviour does, however, not always come from somebody else; sometimes, it comes from within. Therefore, in the next session, we are going to discuss the skill of self-control.

Session 18: Self-Control

AIM, OBJECTIVES, AND OUTLINE

Note to Facilitator. Participant must not only be empowered to handle pressure from outside not to stick to their value-based decisions but also from within. Due to the fact that sexual urges are very strong impulses, it may easily happen that if people do not have good self-control, they will give in to these urges from inside themselves, discarding their value-based decisions and indulging in high-risk sexual behaviour. Therefore, a session is built to strengthen participants' self-control. Participants are taught that it is better to act with an inner locus of control than to let impulses from outside you control your reaction towards the impulse. They are also made aware that sexual self-control does not have to lead to a loss of intimacy in relationships. Participants will discover what can help them exercise self-control so that they will be able to refocus when they are sexually aroused and able to postpone gratification of sexual needs.

Session Aim. By the end of this session, participants will be able to understand that they have the ability to make decisions and through that, exercise control which enable them to exercise responsible or irresponsible social behavior.

Session Objectives. By the end of this session, participants will be able to:
a) Describe what taking control of your situation means.
b) Describe the relationship between self-control and

responsibility.

c) Describe the relationship between self-control and respect.

d) Describe the role that self-control plays in the fight against NEGATIVE MINDSET.

e) Describe ways to conduct sexual self-control in intimate relationships.

Session Outline

Ice-breaker	10 minutes
Group discussion	
Break	
Self-Control and the NEGATIVE MINDSET-epidemic	10 minutes
Self-Control and Intimacy	40 minutes
Personal Action Plan	3 minutes
Conclusion	3 minutes
Total Time	106 minutes

PREPARATION

Preparation by Facilitator
None

Preparation by Participants
None

MATERIALS AND EQUIPMENT
None

ITEM 13-1: ICE-BREAKER

(10 Minutes)

Read the following story:

One day, on an icy cold morning, a young man went hiking in the mountain. On reaching the mountain peak, he came across a rattlesnake – curled up and immobile and very cold. Out of fear the young man stepped back.

The snake spoke up: "Don't be afraid. Please help me, and be my friend. Pick me up and tuck me under your coat, and lay me down on the grass in the village below, where it is warmer and I can survive on my own."

The young man said: "I know you. You are dangerous, and your bite is deadly. Shouldn't have anything to do with you."

Somehow, the snake persuaded the young man to pick it up. He put it under his coat and carried it down to the village.

On reaching the village, the boy took the rattlesnake from under its coat and placed it on the ground.

Just then, the snake bit him and slithered away.

The young man then exclaimed: "But you promised that you would not bite me!"

As it slithers away, it says to the young man, "You knew what I was before you picked me up!"

Ask the group to reflect on their thoughts when they hear that the snake bit the young man. Then, ask them what the moral of the story is and how it can be related to MINDSET.

Lead them in discovering that:

The moral of this story is that you must take responsibility for your actions and not blame others for the consequences of your deeds. If you know that sexual urges can be very strong and lead to a high risk for NEGATIVE MINDSET infection, then don't play with fire.

The young man did not listen to his conscious that said to him: "I shouldn't have anything to do with you." His feelings/emotions overruled his logical thoughts.

ITEM 13-2: Unpacking Self-Control (Exercise 29)

(30 Minutes)

Divide into three groups. Discuss the following questions:

a) Group 1

    i.   If you hear the word "Self-control", what comes to mind?

    ii.   What controls our emotions and behaviour, and what are the factors outside or inside of us?

b) Group 2

    i.   What are the benefits of exercising self-control vs. letting impulses from outside you control you?

    ii.   What are the dangers of letting impulses from outside control you?

c) Group 3

    i.   What role do religion and your conscience play in self-control?

Use *the following to guide the feedback from the groups:* (Use the examples of the electric light of the lecture room and the sun. Show the participants how you switch the light off and on vs. the sun that shines on its own.)

There are two types of people – those who are controlled by their circumstances and those that control their circumstances.

Those who control their circumstances, accept personal responsibility for their reaction to a situation. They make the best of a situation.

People who are controlled by their circumstances, belief

that things happen to them due to things like fate, luck and circumstances, and lies extern from them. They do not accept personal responsibility for their reaction to a situation.

We are confronted daily with situations where we are not in control. Our reaction to such a situation, however, is in our control. In every situation there are decisions to make. It is our right to decide what to do, think, or feel in the situation and to take responsibility for those decisions.

Our perception of a situation determines the degree of excitement or threat that the situation has in it for us. This perception further influences our trust in our own capability to handle the situation.

A person who believes that he is controlled by circumstances may, therefore, experience more stress than a person who believes that he is in control. The person who is controlled by circumstances from outside him will also be less able to handle the stress. This type of person will also experience less work satisfaction than a type of person who sees himself as in control of his decisions and behaviour.

A perception of a situation is formed by what you tell yourself about a situation. If you feed yourself negative information about a situation, it will lead to destructive behaviour from your side. This circle can only be broken if you make a conscious effort to change your personal perception of the situation with positive self-communication.

What does it mean to be controlled by circumstances outside you?
Essentially, you are externally controlled if you assign responsibility for your emotional state in your present moments to someone or something external to yourself.
Thus, *if* you were to be asked the question, "Why do you feel

bad?" and you respond with answers like... "My parents mistreat me," "My friends don't like me," "My luck is down," or "Things just aren't going well" you would be in this external category. Conversely, *if* you were asked why you are so happy, and you responded: "My friends treat me well," "My luck has changed," "Nobody is bugging me," or "She came through for me," you are still in the external frame, assigning responsibility for how you feel to someone or something outside you.

The person who takes control of himself puts the responsibility of how he feels squarely on his own shoulders, and this person is indeed rare in our culture. When asked the same questions, he responds with internally oriented answers such as I tell myself the wrong things, " "I put too much emphasis on what others say," "I worry about what someone else thinks," "I'm not strong enough now to avoid being unhappy, and I worked hard at being happy," "I made things work for me," "I'm telling myself the right things," and "I'm in charge of me, and this is where I choose to be." Thus, one-fourth of the people take responsibility for their own feelings, and three-fourths bestow blame on external sources. Where do you fit in? Virtually all "shoulds" and traditions are imposed by external sources: That is, they come from someone or something outside of you. If you are loaded with should and unable to break conventions which are prescribed by others, then you are in the external bag.

You can never find self-fulfillment if you persist in permitting yourself to be controlled by external forces or persist in thinking that external forces control you. Being effective does not mean eliminating all of the problems in your life. It does mean deciding that you are able to choose your response in any situation. In that way, you make yourself responsible for everything that you experience emotionally.

You are not a robot running your life through a maze filled up with other people's rules and regulations that don't even make sense to you. You can take a sterner look at the rules and begin to exercise some internal control *over* your own thinking feelings, and behaviour.

BREAK

(10 minutes)

ITEM 18-3: SELF-CONTROL AND THE NEGATIVE MINDSET (Exercise 30)

(10 Minutes)

Read the following letter to the participants.

Dear Peter,
It is best that you do not indulge in robbery. Just say "No"!
But I know that you are not capable of controlling yourself and will steal before you reach adulthood.
Therefore, there are some guns and get-away cars that you can steal and not get caught.
But, if you fail and you get arrested, we will find a lawyer who will help you avoid the consequences.

Discuss in plenary the following questions:
What are the similarities between this letter and some approaches to NEGATIVE MINDSET?

Use the following ideas to help guide the feedback from the groups:
A letter with a similar rationale related to NEGATIVE MINDSET may look as follows:

Dear Peter

It is best that you do not indulge in sex outside of marriage. Just say "No"!

But we know that you are not capable of controlling yourself and will have sex before you marry.

Therefore, here are some condoms so you can have sex and NOT get infected.

But, in case you fail, and you do get infected, we will pay for the best medicine to help you avoid the consequences.

This same kind of message with regard to sexual purity is sent out by some NEGATIVE MINDSET programs. It advises people to abstain from premarital sex but have an unspoken attitude that they won't succeed. You must believe that you are capable of controlling your sexual behaviour and capable of making responsible decisions.

TEM 13-4: SELF-CONTROL AND INTIMACY (Exercise 31)

Have the class break into pairs (same-sex would probably be more comfortable). Distribute the following topics amongst the groups. Each pair discuss one of the following topics for 10 minutes afterwards, as many participants as possible will be allowed to share their responses as time allows.

a) What makes it difficult to exercise self-control in an intimate relationship?

b) *Will* sexual self-control necessarily lead to a loss of intimacy in relationships?

c) What role should sexual self-control play in a marriage relationship?

d) What *advice* can you *give* to unmarried couples that will strengthen their capacity to exercise sexual self-control and that will lead to refocus when sexually aroused and to the postponement of gratification of needs?

e) What is your opinion of the role of masturbation in sexual self-control?

f) What can a married person do to exercise self-control when he/she starts to feel attracted to somebody else at work?

Use the following ideas *to* help guide the feedback from the groups and to integrate their previous learning:

Self-control is *very* important to *live* a NEGATIVE MINDSET-free life. To be able to exercise this self-control, it is necessary that you have a clear idea of who you are and what your values are. You will need self-confidence and assertiveness to turn down unwanted sex.

When you act with self-control, you will have time to contemplate whether an action is in line with the Golden Rule or whether you are not doing unto another that you don't want them to do unto you.

ITEM 13-5: PERSONAL ACTION PLAN

(3 Minutes)

Write on your personal commitment sheet what you intend to do to increase yourself control and ability to act with self-control. Will you walk the talk?

ITEM 13-6: CONCLUSION

Self-control is a very important skill if you want to stay true to the value of the Golden Rule ("Do unto others as you want them to do unto you"). It enables you to stick to your values in difficult circumstances. It is needed when you want to act responsibly and when you want to respect others. Self-control is possible when you make a commitment to sound, ethically-based decisions.

A specific situation in which self-control is needed is a

conflict situation. People without self-control in conflict situations can ruin relationships permanently. This can be avoided if they have the necessary conflict management skills. This leads to sequential breaks in relationships, which is a breathing space for the spread of the NEGATIVE MINDSET. Therefore, in the next section, we address the topic of conflict handling.

Session 19: Conflict Management and Resolution

AIM, OBJECTIVES, AND OUTLINE

Note to Facilitator. Apart from implementing value-based decisions through assertiveness and self-control, strong relationships are another cornerstone to reducing the risk of NEGATIVE MINDSET infection. Therefore, a module is put in place to teach participants how to build relationships based on sound values. A basic skill that is needed to build these strong relationships is the knowledge of how to handle conflicts. In order to live out the values that a person has decided on, he/she will have to be able to confront other people with his/her decisions. This may lead to conflict. How this is done in such a way that the relationship does not deteriorate is the topic in this session on conflict handling.

Session Aim. By the end of this session, participants will be able to handle conflict as part of spiritual, ethical and moral conduct. This will enable them to conduct more permanent relationships.

Session Objectives

By the end of this session, participants will be able to:
   a) Describe the steps in healthy conflict resolution.
   b) Identify different ways people handle conflict.
   c) Describe the role of forgiving in conflict management.

Session Outline

a) Ice-Breaker:
b) Conflict Resolution steps
c) Tips for Conflict Handling
d) Forgiving
e) Values and Conflict Handling
f) Personal Action Plan

PREPARATION

Preparation by Facilitator
None

Preparation by Participants
None

MATERIALS AND EQUIPMENT

Copies of different styles of conflict handling for each participant.

ITEM 14-1: ICE-BREAKER

(15 Minutes)

Request two participants of t h e opposite gender to role-play the following scenario.

A married man was tested and was found to have NEGATIVE MINDSET+. This led to mistrust between him and his wife. One was accusing the other of bringing the disease into the family.

Ask the group to discuss what is necessary to solve this problem. Tell the group that there are six generic steps to solve the problem. Take the steps one by one, and with the group's participation, using a flip chart, come to a solution.

The following are generic steps that help to solve conflicts.

a) Define the problem and make sure that there are no misconceptions.
b) Brainstorm possible solutions.
c) Consider and evaluate all the possible solutions and suggestions.
d) Choose the most acceptable or suitable solutions.
e) Support each other and put the solution into practice.
f) Reconsider and evaluate.

ITEM 14-2: TIPS FOR CONFLICT HANDLING

(15 Minutes)

Ask the following question in plenary:
What tips can you give to each other on how to handle conflict?

List their responses and then enrich them with some of the following:
a) Listen to what the other person says.
b) Do not withdraw.
c) Do not become defensive.
d) Do not act as if you do not care.
e) Admit that there is a difference in opinion.
f) Do not avoid conflict.
g) Choose a time that works for both parties to sort out the problem.
h) Be sensitive to the other person's feelings.
i) Determine if there is nothing else that has nothing to do with the problem that really bothers the other person.
j) Do not interrupt.
k) Place yourself in the other person's situation.
l) Reflect on the person and what the person says in order

to find out whether you understand him/her correctly.

m) Avoid "You" messages: "You have done this; you are lazy, etc."

n) Send "I" messages: "I feel sad when you... "

o) Identify the specific problem.

p) Tackle the problem and not each other.

q) Do not involve other people, family, parents, in-laws, or friends that have nothing to do with the problem: "Yes, you are just like your mother."

r) Be specific. Do not generalize.

s) Avoid words like "always" and "never".

t) Stay with the present; do not go back to old fights.

u) Investigate the possible solutions. Choose the best option through a process of elimination.

v) Do self-introspection: "What is my share in this conflict?" "Can I change my behaviour or attitude to help solve the problem?"

w) Avoid drama – taking off your wedding ring, burning your marriage certificate, etc.

x) Forgive.

y) Do not defend yourself – be an adult and admit if you have made a fault.

z) Be prepared to say sorry.

aa) Show that you still love your partner despite the conflict.

ITEM 14-3: FORGIVING (Exercise 32)

(15 Minutes)

Divide into two groups. Each group discuss one of the following topics for ten minutes. Give feedback for five minutes.

a) What *is* the role of forgiving in reconciliation and in the building of lifelong quality relationships? Take into consideration the statement: 'To make mistakes is human, to forgive divine."

b) What role does forgiving play in a NEGATIVE MINDSET-infected person's capacity to cope with his/her infection?

Use the following ideas to help guide the feedback from the groups:

Important elements of the road to forgiveness include the following:

a) Estrangement
   i. The victim experience injury that alienates him from the offender.
b) Healing of the inner self
   i. A rediscovery of the humanity of the offender must take place.
   ii. The right to get even must be surrendered.
   iii. The victim's feelings about the offender must be changed.
c) Reconciliation
   i. It can only start if healing took place in the victim. The victim has worked through his/her pain.
   ii. Although forgiveness is always unconditional, reconciliation is conditional. One such condition is honesty.
d) Hope
   i. Hope follows after forgiveness and reconciliation.
   ii. Hope creates the possibility to realize ideals in the future (e.g. lifelong partnerships).

Remind them that to forgive others are in line with the Golden Rule. Ask them what makes it difficult for them to forgive others?

ITEM 14-4: VALUES AND CONFLICT HANDLING (Exercise 33)
(25 Minutes)

Request them to stay in the same subgroups and discuss the following for 10 minutes. Give feedback for five minutes.

- How does Ubuntu and the values of love, responsibility, respect, integrity, and fairness manifest in sound conflict handling?'

- What are the implications if I do not have sound conflict management skills?

ITEM 14-5: PERSONAL ACTION PLAN

(3 Minutes)

Write down on your personal commitment sheet what you intend to do in future to improve your way of conflict handling. Will you walk the talk?

ITEM 14-6: CONCLUSION

(2 Minutes)

The ability to handle conflict has a serious impact on the quality of relationships in our society. People who have sound conflict handling skills are able to engage in more permanent relationship, and therefore contribute to a more stable environment, in which the spread of NEGATIVE MINDSET can be less.

If you are committed to your convictions, say to yourself: "Because I believe what I believe in terms of values, I will handle conflict in a way that will not compromise my values. I will act in accordance with the Golden Rule in all my conflict handling."

In the next sessions we are going to discuss how relationships are formed that are permanent. If a person knows how to handle conflict and how to build relationships, he/she will be ensured of a stable network of relationships that will enable him/her to live a NEGATIVE MINDSET-risk free life.

Module V
Relationships

Session 20: Friendships

AIM, OBJECTIVES, AND OUTLINE

Note to Facilitator. In the previous session we have discussed the importance of conflict handling in the maintenance of strong relationships. This session is built to make participants aware of how the development of friendships takes place. How are friendships built? How does it develop from a friendship to an intimate one?

Relationship? What is the place of sex in intimacy? Is abstinence outside marriage a dream?

Session Aim. By the end of this session, participants will be able to form friendships in such a way that there is no risk of NEGATIVE MINDSET.

Session Objectives. By the end of this session, participants will be able to:
a) Distinguish between genuine and artificial friendship.
b) Describe what marriage entails.
c) Describe what the danger zones are if a person wants to abstain from sexual intercourse until marriage.

Session Outline

The progression in friendship	30 minutes
Break	5 minutes
Icarus and the wax wings	5 minutes
Group discussions: Abstinence	35 minutes
Personal Action Plan	3 minutes
Conclusion	2 minutes
Total Time	80 minutes

ITEM 15-1: THE PROGRESSION IN FRIENDSHIP (Exercise 34)
(30 Minutes)

Divide into five groups. Tell them that the following discussion is about the different stages of true friendships. Request them to discuss the following for ten minutes. Thereafter, give feedback.

a) <u>Group 1</u>: What are the characteristics of a true friendship? How do you develop a genuine friendship?

b) <u>Group 2</u>: What are the warning signs of an artificial friendship?

c) <u>Group 3</u>: How do we develop genuine friendships? What must we do from our side?

d) <u>Group 4</u>: What changes when a friendship changes into a relationship? What happens? What does it mean to fall in love?

e) <u>Group 5</u>: When is it time to marry?

Use the following ideas to help guide the feedback from the groups:

The characteristics of true friendship are that it is value-based:

Trust, honesty, faithfulness, sharing, unselfish love,

tolerance, understanding, sensitivity, politeness, openness, openness to correction, sacrifice, compromise, reliability, and freedom. (All of these are in line with the spirit of Ubuntu and the Golden Rule).

Warning signs of artificial friendship:
Pretence, disloyalty, unfaithfulness, exploitation, manipulation, insensitivity, gossip, lies, disobedience, unhappiness, selfishness, jealousy, boasting, backstabbing, secretiveness, annoyance, and dominance. (All this is not in line with the spirit of Ubuntu and the Golden Rule)

Things that we can do to develop genuine friendships:
Work on all the things mentioned above that are the characteristics of a genuine friendship. Make friendships a priority. One step at a time. Do things together.

Signs that a friendship changes into a relationship:
There is extra love and special attention, intimacy starts, and passion comes *in*. *You* start to share intimate things with the person that you would not share with other people. You get personal. You open up to a new level. You begin to hold hands, kiss and cuddle. You become vulnerable because the relationship *is* special. You can be hurt. You take responsibility for the other person. The other person brings out the best in you.

When is the time ready to marry?
When you have peace *in* your heart that this is the one that you want to spend your whole life, you commit yourself because *you* just know "this is the one". When there is stability in the relationship, when you know each other long enough that both are unable to pretend in front of the other one. This does

not happen in three months' time when you feel completely comfortable in this relationship. When you are inseparable, you are able to laugh and cry together. When there is cognitive (logic), conative (decision) and emotive harmony in you about the other person:

Cognitive level: Logically it makes sense – I can live with this person for the rest of my life.

Conative level (Motivational level): I want to marry this person.

BREAK

(5 Minutes)

Emotional level: I feel attracted to this person.

ITEM 15-2: ICARUS AND THE WAX WINGS

(Taken From Crossroads Program P19-7)

Read the following story to the group. Afterwards, ask them to reflect on what their emotions and thoughts were when they heard the story and what lesson they think can be learnt from it.

King Minos had cruelly imprisoned Icarus and his father, Darius, in a tower. Darius was a skillful builder and inventor, and it was the king's command that Darius invented many wonderful things for his pleasure.

Darius determined that he and Icarus would escape the tower by flying away. Summoning all the secrets of his craft, he set to work constructing a pair of wings. Little by little, he gathered a great pile of feathers of all sizes. He fastened them together with thread and moulded them with wax. Finally, he had two great wings, like those of the seagulls. He tied them to his shoulders and, waving his arms, rose into the air, gliding and soaring on the currents.

Next, he built a second pair of wings for Icarus and taught him how to ride the air currents, climbing in circles and hanging in the winds. They practised together until Icarus was ready.

Finally, the day came when the winds were just right. Father and son strapped on their wings and prepared to fly home.

"Remember all I've told you," Darius said, "Above all, remember you must not fly too high. If you do, the heat of the sun will melt the wax, and your wings will fall apart. Stay close to me, and you'll be fine."

Up they rose, the boy and his father. At first, the flight seemed terrible to both Darius and Icarus, but gradually, they grew accustomed to riding among the clouds, and they lost their fear. Icarus felt the wind fill his wings and lift him higher and higher, and he began to sense a freedom he had never known before. He looked down with great excitement at all the islands they passed, their people, and the broad blue sea spread out beneath him, dotted with the white sails of ships. He soared higher and higher, forgetting his father's warning. He forgot everything in the world but the joy of flying.

"Come back!" Darius called frantically, "You're flying too high! Remember the sun! Come down! Come down!"

But Icarus thought of nothing but his own excitement. He longed to fly as close as he could to the heavens. Nearer and nearer, he came to the sun, and slowly, his wings began to soften. One by one, the feathers began to fall and scatter in the air, and suddenly, the wax melted completely. Icarus felt himself falling. He fluttered his arms as fast as he could, but no feathers remained to hold the air. He cried out for his father, but it was too late – with a scream, he fell from his lofty height and plunged into the sea, disappearing beneath the waves forever.

Reflect on this story by saying that it is important to plan your relationship:

You must remember that any good and healthy relationship needs to grow and develop. If you decide you want to wait for sex until you marry, then you must allow space in your physical relationship for that natural development.

The problem is that very often, you may say you want to wait for sex, but then, within weeks of starting your relationship, you may have allowed your physical relationship to progress to just short of having sex – touching each other's sexual organs, heavy petting, etc. Then, it becomes very difficult for both of you to stick to your decisions in waiting for sex.

It is also important to remember that men are different from women in the way that they become sexually aroused. With women, It Is a slower, more even process. Very often, women do not realize this difference. Girls would, for instance, allow the boys to touch or caress their breasts. They might still be able to resist the pressure to progress towards sex, but at that stage, it is very difficult for the guy to think straight.

ITEM 15-3: GROUP DISCUSSION: ABSTINENCE

(35 Minutes)

Divide into five groups. Discuss the following for 10 minutes, and then let every group give 5 minutes of feedback.

a) <u>Group 1:</u> Is it still an achievable goal to maintain abstinence until marriage? What factors make *it* difficult?
b) <u>Group 2:</u> What is your religion's view on abstinence before marriage?
c) <u>Group 3:</u> What are the benefits of abstinence until marriage?
d) <u>Group 4:</u> What implications does the story of "Icarus and

the wax wings" have for dating? How close is too close? What are the danger zones if a person wants to abstain?

e) <u>Group 5</u>: Discuss the following in terms of sound values and the NEGATIVE MINDSET – risk. "In my tradition, before you marry, a woman must have a baby. You test drive before you buy a car."

Use the following ideas to help guide the feedback from the groups:

a) Abstinence offers a number of advantages.
b) It eliminates the risk of unplanned pregnancy.
c) It requires no visits to clinics or supplies of contraceptives.
d) It protects you from sexually transmitted infections.
e) It is available at any time.
f) The only disadvantage of abstinence is that it requires strong motivation, self-control, and commitment.'

ITEM 15-4: PERSONAL ACTION PLAN

Write on your personal commitment sheet what you intend to do in future to increase the level of building your friendships on a basis of values.

Will you walk the talk?

ITEM 15-5: CONCLUSION

(12 Minutes)

Summarize. We have discussed the difference between true and artificial friendships, and have also discussed the risks for the person who has chosen to abstain until marriage.

The story of Icarus and the Wax Wings tells us that we tend to think that we can control ourselves and stop ourselves just in time from going one step too far. Unfortunately, when we play life so close to the edge, we sometimes can't avoid getting burned. When life itself is at stake, a wise person does not try to see how close he can get to the edge. With NEGATIVE MINDSET/AIDS being such a deadly disease, the wise person will stick to sound values to ensure he/she and his/her family are saved from it.

Therefore, say to yourself: "Because I believe what I believe, I will treat all my friends according to my values of always acting in love, being responsible, being fair, with integrity and respect. I will stay true to the spirit of Ubuntu and the Golden Rule".

In the next session, we will discuss the issue of a relationship that has developed into a relationship with a life partner. How do I ensure that it stays a partnership for life, in which there will be no need for extra-marital sex?

SESSION 3: INTRODUCING VALUES

ITEM 3-1: WHAT ARE VALUES AND HOW DO THEY INFLUENCE OUR LIVES? (Exercise 3)

Divide the group into subgroups of 4-5 people. Ask them to read through the following exercise: (Exercise: Crocodile River). Give them 7 minutes to complete the reading.

Characters: HECTOR, the hero; ANNALINE, the angel; SINBAD, the sailor; BARNEY, the brave; and WILFRED, the wise.

Once upon a time, there was a young couple, Hector and Anneline, who were very much in love; they lived on opposite sides of a wide, crocodile-infested river which was spanned only by a footbridge. They visited each other every day, and being f1_rm believers in sex after marriage, they spent many happy evenings together playing *Scrabble, Monopoly* and Ludo. They had great plans to be married sometime in the not-too-distant future.

One day, a *terrible* storm arose, and the *river* flooded, washing the little footbridge between their houses away, so they had no way to see each other. Annaline became lonelier and *lonelier,* longing to see her Hector. So, she lost weight and became thinner and thinner. Finally, she decided to plan to get over to see Hector, so she went *downriver* to Sinbad, the sailor, who had a boat, and she asked Sinbad to row her across the river to see Hector. Sinbad agreed to do so on condition that Annaline have sex with *him* first.

Anneline was horrified, refused, and rushed home again. After a couple of days, she again became so *lonely* that she went to see an old man in a cave in the hills, known as *Wilfred* the Wise. She told her story to him, telling him about Sinbad and seeking his advice on what to do. Wilfred listened carefully to all she had to say but would give her no advice at all as to what she should do.

Again, Anneline wrestled, but finally gave way, went to Sinbad and agreed to spend the night with him if he would row her over to see Hector. Sinbad kept his side of the bargain and when Hector saw Annaline running along the road to his gate, he was overjoyed to see her and held her closely in his arms. Annaline confessed to Hector how she had missed him and longed for him and what it was that she had done to reach him again.

When Hector, who was a very moral and good person, heard Annaline's tale, he flew into a rage and flung her from him, saying that she had betrayed him and their principles.

Annaline fell to the ground, weeping bitterly.

Just then, Barney the brave, who had witnessed the scene, Cam riding up on his White horse, gently scooped

Annaline from the ground after punching Hector for his rude behaviour, put her on his horse and rode away into the sunset with Anneline Wrapped closely in his arms.

After the participants have read the above passage, ask them to do the following for 15 minutes. Allow 10 minutes for feedback:
   a) Rate the five people's behaviour from the most acceptable to the least acceptable according to the value system that is important TO YOU.
   b) Thereafter, discuss amongst each other what you understand under the term "Value".
   c) Lastly, discuss which values you think are necessary to strengthen the fight against NEGATIVE MINDSET.

Use the following ideas to help guide the feedback from the groups:
A 'Value" is a *personal belief.*
It is a personal belief that *certain behaviours are the ones we prefer.*
Values direct our thoughts, decisions and behaviour.
We use our values as a measuring tool for *measuring standards of behaviour.*
Your values are your personal *standard of conduct.* We use it to evaluate our own behaviour.
Your values are also your measure of assessing the standard of conduct *in others.*

We use our values to condemn, justify or legitimise behaviour.

Many factors can lead to us acting in accordance with our personal values, e.g. lack of self-confidence, group pressure, and strong urges. When we do not act in accordance with our own values, we may have guilty feelings or feelings of failure.

We receive our values from our environment, especially from our parents, when we are small.

The values of different people differ.

In the fight against NEGATIVE MINDSET, we cannot be neutral about values.

NEGATIVE MINDSET prevention is linked with responsible behaviour. Responsible behaviour has to do with what you or others regard as up to standard or as right and wrong.

ITEM 3-2: THE VALUE FRAMEWORK OF THIS COURSE

(15 Minutes)

Explain* to *the group that all the values that a person or group of persons adhere to can be called the value framework of this person or group of persons.

There are different value frameworks that a person can operate within, e.g. religious frameworks (Christianity, Hinduism, etc.), philosophical frameworks (pragmatist, humanist, etc.), and cultural frameworks (Ubuntu, Western, Eastern, etc.).

As everybody operates from a value framework, it is impossible to talk about values without doing it from a value framework.

This course has the following value framework:

The *core/common values* vital for the protection and survival of societies, which can be found in most religions.

Those values are grouped together in the cultural value framework of *"Ubuntu"*.

The **Golden Rule** of "Do unto others as you want to be done unto:"

We know that the foundation of values lies deep. As we

said, values stem from religious, philosophical, cultural and other convictions. The values are like pillars built on these convictions. Our whole life, all our behaviour rests on these values and flows from them.

There are many values, but for this course the following core values were selected: Love, Responsibility, Fairness, Integrity, Respect and Professionalism.

Behaviour											
Religious, Cultural and Other Convictions											

ITEM 3-3: PERSONAL ACTION PLAN

(3 Minutes)

a. Write down in the space allowed next to questions 1 and *2* on your personal commitment sheet:

b. How would you label the religious, philosophical or cultural value framework that you operate from?

c. Which specific values are very important to you?

ITEM 3-4: IMPORTANT OR NOT IMPORTANT CUSTOMS? (Exercise 4)

(40 Minutes)

Divide into two groups. Ask the groups to discuss the following subjects for 20 minutes. Reserve *20* minutes for feedback. Summarize after the feedback. (The aim of this exercise is to give the facilitator insight into the values of the participants).

What importance do you as a group attach to the following? What meaning does it have for you?

a) Group 1

 i. Marriage?

 ii. Sex?

b) <u>Group 2</u>
  i.   Chastity?
  ii.   Abstaining from sex outside a permanent relationship?
  iii. Virginity?

Use the following ideas to help guide the feedback from the groups:

Sex feelings are normal and real, and no one should be embarrassed for having them. However, acting on the basis of these feelings alone can turn sex from a very good thing to a bad thing, meaning that it may have bad consequences.

Sex involves all dimensions of a person. Therefore, there are mental, emotional, social and spiritual consequences when I enter into a sexual relationship.

In all major religions, sex is seen as something that belongs within the borders of marriage. Virginity, abstinence and chastity outside the borders of marriage are highly valued by all major religions.

ITEM 3-5: RELIGION AND VALUES (Exercise: 5)

(20 Minutes)

Discuss the following in groups:

What role does religion play in the forming of values?

What does your religion/ethical framework tell you about values that are preferred with regard to sex? Why would the Supreme Being (God) prefer these values?

Which different categories of values can you distinguish in today's society on the topic of sex inside and outside the boundaries of marriage?

Use the following ideas to help guide the feedback from the groups:

In our society, the following categories can be identified:

a) People who believe in the holiness of marriage believe that sex belongs in marriage. Abstinence before marriage and faithfulness in marriage are important. (Traditional religious viewpoint)

b) People who do not value marriage as such but believe that sex must take place in an environment of values, love, respect, integrity and responsibility. In this group, abstinence before marriage is not a requirement, but faithfulness in permanent relationships is important.

c) People do not see sex as something holy which can be enjoyed wherever and with whomever they like. The individual is a free person to do as he/she likes.

ITEM 3-6: CULTURE AND NEGATIVE MINDSET (Exercise: 6)

(25 Minutes)

Discuss the following in three groups for 10 minutes, and give feedback for 15 minutes:

a) Which cultural values or practices in the South African Community do you think contribute to the spread of NEGATIVE MINDSET, and which contribute to the curbing of the spread of NEGATIVE MINDSET?

b) Which practices in your environment do you see as high-risk practices, and which would you like to warn your children against?

c) What are your feelings about Ubuntu?

Use the following ideas to help guide the discussions of the groups:

Explore the role of cultural practices like politics, lobola, secular government, initiation schools, etc.

When the group give feedback on Ubuntu, tell them that we will regularly come back to this concept and give the following definition:

'Ubuntu" means to be human, to value the good of the community above self-interest, to strive to help other people in the spirit of service, to show respect to others and to be honest and trustworthy. "I am because of others".

ITEM 3-7: CONCLUSION

(3 Minutes)

We have now discovered that we all have personal values that direct our behaviour. These values form part of a value framework that has as its foundation religious, philosophical, cultural and other convictions. "Because I believe, what I believe, I want to follow these values." We use these values to measure the standard of behavior in ourselves and in others. We are going to concentrate on some values during this course to measure whether certain behavior will help in the prevention of NEGATIVE MINDSET or not.

Right through this course, you will be confronted with the question: "Do you walk the talk?" This means: Do you act according to the values that you say you have chosen? In particular, the next question will be a refrain. Are you loyal to the Golden Rule of doing unto others as you want them to do unto you?

ITEM 3-8: INTRODUCING THE NEXT SESSION

(13 Minutes)

Inform the group: We have now explored the importance of value-driven lifestyles. In the next session, we are going to explore your self-identity, who you are and what your dreams are. We need to stand still on this, as it is important to know.

Session 23: A Higher Spiritual Authority Demanding Value-Driven Lives

AIM, OBJECTIVES, AND OUTLINE

Note to Facilitators. The module on relationships ends with a session with a person's relationship with a higher spiritual authority or "God". It is impossible to discuss value-driven lives without discussing the influence of a relationship with a higher spiritual authority, or "God". What implication does the participant's relationship with this higher spiritual authority have for the risk of HIV infection?

Session Aim. By the end of this session, participants have reflected on their "Higher Spiritual Authority"/ God's expectations of them in terms of a value-based life.

Session Objectives. By the end of this session, participants will be able to:
a) Identify where their lives are not in line with their religious convictions.
b) Commit themselves to a life in line with their religious convictions.

Session Outline.

Introspection	20 minutes
Personal Action Plan	5 minutes

PREPARATION

Preparation by Facilitator
None

Preparation by Participants
None

ITEM 18-1: INTROSPECTION (Exercise: 41)

Request all participants to go as individuals and find a place where they can be on their own. Tell them to take a piece of paper with them, as well as their personal commitment sheets. Give them 15 minutes to reflect on their own on the following questions. They must write their responses down on the paper. Let them thereafter fill in the questions on their personal commitment sheets.

a) What does my Creator expect from me in terms of a value-driven life? (For example, He expects me to believe, to be obedient, not to harm other people, to care for other people, and to live a pure life.) How do these expectations relate to what is written on my personal commitment sheet?

b) What is my response to those expectations? Do I meet those expectations? Is my interaction with other people, my daily life and my sexual behaviour in line with those expectations?

c) In those cases where my life is not in line with those expectations, what can I do to bring it in line with it?

d) Read the pledge that is the last item on the personal commitment sheet and decide whether you are ready to commit yourself to signing it.

When sending the participants away to go and do introspection, tell them: ·

We often tend to separate what we believe from how we live from day to day and from how we interact with other people. We say that we believe in a certain religion and its values, but we do not act according to it. With this type of behavior we tend to harm others and ourselves. Therefore go and do introspection and decide what you will do to get your life in line with your spiritual commitment.

ITEM 18-2: PERSONAL ACTION PLAN

Write on your personal commitment sheet what you intend to do in future to increase your level of being true to your commitment to the values expected from you by your Higher Spiritual Authority/God.

Will you walk the talk?

Module VI
Commitment

Session 24: Reflection, Pledging and Celebrating

AIM, OBJECTIVES, AND OUTLINE

Note to Facilitator. The course ends with a session where participants reflect on what they have experienced, and they are given the opportunity to make a pledge to live a value-based life and this commitment is then celebrated.

Session Aim. By the end of this session, participants will have reflected on the content of this course and pledged to an ethical, value-driven lifestyle.

Session Objectives. By the end of this session, participants will be able to:
   a) Reflect on what they have learned during the programme.
   b) Commit themselves to a value-driven lifestyle.

Session Outline

Reflection	10 minutes
Feedback	10 minutes
Drawing	20 minutes
Personal Commitment Sheets	10 minutes
Success Stories	10 minutes
Celebration	60 minutes
Total Time	120 minutes

PREPARATION

Preparation by Facilitator
- a) Prepare certificates.
- b) Organise snacks.
- c) Organise VIP to hand out certificates and say a few words.

Preparation by Participants
None

MATERIALS AND EQUIPMENT
- a) Snacks Certificates
- b) Pens to make a drawing Flip chart.

Session 25: Living the Values: Reflections, Commitments, and Celebrations

ITEM 19-1: REFLECTION (Exercise: 42)

Request the group to go back to the table of contents. Refresh their minds quickly on what was done in the different sessions.

Ask them to choose one of the following slogans which describe what they have learnt during the course the best. Ask them to give a reason why they have chosen it. They may also develop an own slogan.

"Sex belongs within marriage."

"Virginity is a special gift, and it's wonderful to give it to your life partner."

"True love waits."

"Proud to be an unmarried virgin."

"'Safe sex' really means 'No sex' outside marriage."

"Abstinence and Be Faithful is today's AIDS Vaccine."

"You have the final choice. Choose right -choose life."

"Faithfulness is *cool!*"

"Beware of peer pressure – it could cost your life."

"One partner for *life.*"

"Treasure your life-stop AIDS."

"Treasure your *family* – Keep AIDS away."

"Do unto others as you want them to do unto you."

"Integrity – Do I have what it takes?" "Respect – stands the test of *time.*"

"Be fair – *live* and let live!"

"Be responsible – bad *decisions* are irreversible."
"Love is...not killing your family!"
19-4

ITEM 19-2: FEEDBACK

Divide into four groups. Ask the participants to discuss the following in the groups and then give feedback to the plenary:
    a) What was positive about the course?
    b) What was negative?
    c) What advice can they give to make the course better for future participants?
Request that one person be the scribe and write down their responses.

ITEM 19-3: DRAWING

Let every group take a piece of flip chart paper and give them ten minutes to draw a picture/symbol which summarizes what they have learned this past week. Let them share it with the rest of the groups.

ITEM 19-4: PERSONAL COMMITMENT SHEETS

Let every person take his personal commitment sheet and read through all that they have written down during the course. Tell them that during the celebration, they are going to have the opportunity to voluntarily make a pledge where they can commit themselves to executing their personal commitments and living a value-based lifestyle.

ITEM 19-5: DEPART TO THE PLACE WHERE THE CELEBRATION WILL TAKE PLACE

Start by welcoming guests.

ITEM 19-6: SUCCESS STORIES

Give an opportunity to those who want to tell what the course has meant to them and what they intend to do with the knowledge and skills which they have acquired.

ITEM 19-7: CELEBRATION

Have a ceremony where each one wants to pledge and sign a pledge certificate. The wording of the pledge on the Certificate can be something like the following:

<table>
<tr><td>

By the grace of my Creator, I, _____________________, make a pledge to Him, Myself, my family and my (future)

Spouse to uphold a high spiritual and ethical lifestyle and to keep myself sexually pure, mentally pure.

I made this pledge after attending the program, "Combat negative mindset through Ethical and Spiritual

Conduct" over the period _____________ to _____________ at _____________ .

_______________   _______________   _______________

My signature   Program Leader   Date

</td></tr>
</table>

Begin the pledging ceremony by letting everybody read the pledge loudly.

Prepare a table where participants sign a pledge.

Let an important person congratulate them after signing the certificate.

Give an opportunity to the important person to say a few words.

Have some champagne to celebrate their decision to live a value-based life.

Afterwards, provide snacks.

REFERENCES

1. A.M. Educational Consultants. (1999). *Life skills and HIV/AIDS education program: Teacher's resource guide for grades 1-7*. Pretoria, South Africa.
2. Department of Education. (2002, March 25-27). *Beyond advocacy* [Conference session]. Department of Education Conference, Pretoria, South Africa.
3. Edward-Meyer, D. (2002). *HIV/AIDS program: Africa wellness: Sexual health education, AIDS, life skills training and help* [Unpublished program].
4. Edwards, D., & Louw, N. (1998). *Outcomes-based sexuality education*. Pretoria, South Africa.
5. Greyling, C. (2002). *Old Mutual's "I have hope" AIDS program: Presenter's manual*. Stellenbosch, South Africa.
6. Marks, E. (Ed.). (1995). *Life at the crossroads: An educational curriculum program from Youth at the Cross*. Orlando, FL, USA.
7. South African Military Health Service. (2001, May). *Education Officers' HIV training participant's manual*. Pretoria, South Africa: SAMHS.
8. UNAIDS. (1999). *Sexual behavioural change for HIV: Where have theories taken us?* Geneva, Switzerland.
9. Van Niekerk, A. (Ed.). (n.d.). *AIDS in context: A South African perspective*.

Contact Persons: Rev. Jongikhaya Siwali
Email: jongisiwal@gmail.com /www.lightofgodfellowship.com
Mobile: 0849756357
Course Aims:

Aim of the course is to show that without Spirituality and Ethics disciplines it is difficult to make it in life. So, this speaks of them employing a positive mindset founded in those disciples and we then practically show it by this product.